Yoga for Beginners

100 Yoga Poses to
Calm the Mind, Relieve Stress,
Strengthen the Body, and
Increase Flexibility

Noah Miller

Copyrights

All rights reserved © 2017 by Noah Miller. No part of this publication or the information in it may be quoted from or reproduced in any form by means such as printing, scanning, photocopying, or otherwise without prior written permission of the copyright holder.

Disclaimer and Terms of Use

Efforts has been made to ensure that the information in this book is accurate and complete. However, the author and the publisher do not warrant the accuracy of the information, text, and graphics contained within the book due to the rapidly changing nature of science, research, known and unknown facts, and internet. The author and the publisher do not hold any responsibility for errors, omissions, or contrary interpretation of the subject matter herein. This book is presented solely for motivational and informational purposes only

ISBN: 978-1985024632

Printed in the United States

Contents

CONTENTS	3
INTRODUCTION	1
WHAT IS YOGA?	3
Well then, what is yoga?	3
TYPES OF YOGA	7
A BRIEF HISTORY OF YOGA	9
THE PHILOSOPHY BEHIND YOGA	11
THE HEALTH BENEFITS OF YOGA	13
100 YOGA POSES FOR BEGINNERS	17
GUIDELINES FOR YOGA PRACTICE	19
BASIC YOGA POSES	21
Staff Pose	21
Half Lotus Pose	23
Seated Mountain Pose	25
Hero Pose	27
Half Squat Pose	29
Tiger Pose	31
One Handed Tiger Pose	33
Lion Pose	35
Bound Angle Pose	37
One Legged Boat Pose	39
Wide Angle Seated Forward Bend	41
Half Bow Pose	43
Crocodile Pose	45
Thread the Needle Pose	47
Eye of the Needle Pose	49
Happy Baby Pose	51
Mountain Pose	53
Half Wheel Pose	55
Standing Spinal Twist Pose	57
Lateral Half Moon Pose	59
Double Angle Pose	61
Gate Pose	63
Goddess Pose	65

Corpse Pose	67
Eight-Limbed Pose	69
BASIC POSES FOR STRENGTHENING THE ARMS	**71**
	71
Reverse Table Top Pose	71
Cobra Pose	73
Plank Pose	75
INTERMEDIATE POSES FOR STRENGTHENING ARMS	**77**
Dolphin Plank Pose	77
Upward Facing Dog Pose	79
Elevated Lotus Pose	81
BASIC POSES FOR STRETCHING AND STRENGTHENING THE LEGS	**83**
Chair Pose	85
Standing Forward Bend	87
Tree Pose	89
Downward Facing Dog Pose	91
High Lunge Pose	93
Warrior Pose I	95
Warrior Pose II	97
Garland Pose	99
INTERMEDIATE POSES FOR STRENGTHENING LEGS	**101**
Intense Side Stretch	101
Revolved Side Angle Pose	103
Warrior Pose III	105
BASIC POSES FOR STRENGTHENING THE SHOULDERS	**107**
Big Toe Pose	107
Bharadvaja's Twist	109
Cow Pose	111
Cat Pose	113
Bow Pose	115
Camel Pose	117
INTERMEDIATE POSES FOR STRENGTHENING THE SHOULDERS	**119**
Side Plank Pose	119
Eagle Pose	121
BASIC POSES FOR STRENGTHENING THE CORE	**123**
Boat Pose	125

Locust Pose	127
Half Prayer Twist	129
Dolphin Pose	131
One-Legged Down Dog Pose	133
Extended Triangle Pose	134
INTERMEDIATE POSES FOR STRENGTHENING THE CORE	**137**
Tiptoe Pose	137
One-Legged Bridge Pose	139
Four-Limbed Staff Pose	141
BASIC POSES FOR THE HIPS	**143**
Easy Pose	143
Half Lord of the Fishes Pose	145
Child's Pose	147
Bound Angle Pose	149
Reclining Bound Angle Pose	151
Cow Face Pose	152
INTERMEDIATE POSES FOR THE HIPS	**155**
Half Pigeon Pose	155
Extended Hand-To-Big-Toe Pose	157
YOGA FOR VARIOUS HEALTH CONDITIONS	**159**
YOGA FOR HEADACHE	**161**
Lotus Pose	161
Thunderbolt Pose	163
Extended Puppy Pose	165
Seated Forward Bend	167
Bridge Pose	169
Upside-Down Seal Yoga Pose	171
Fire Log Pose	173
YOGA FOR INDIGESTION AND CONSTIPATION	**175**
Wind Relieving Pose	175
Half Tortoise Pose	177
Head to Knee Pose	179
Revolved Triangle Pose	181
Half Camel Pose	183
Half Plough Pose	185
YOGA FOR ASTHMA	**187**

THE PSYCHIC UNION POSE	187
SHOULDER STAND	189
FISH POSE	191
YOGA FOR NECK PAIN	**193**
EASY POSE WITH TWIST	193
SEATED EAGLE POSE	195
TWISTED POSE	197
YOGA FOR BACK PAIN	**199**
SPHINX POSE	199
RABBIT POSE	201
UPWARD PLANK POSE	203
YOGA FOR MENSTRUAL DISORDERS AND MENOPAUSE	**205**
HALF MOON POSE	205
EXTENDED SIDE ANGLE POSE	207
RECLINING HERO POSE	209
RECLINING HAND-TO-BIG-TOE POSE	211
YOGA FOR RELIEVING GAS	**213**
SUPINE SPINAL TWIST	213
WIDE-LEGGED FORWARD BEND POSE	215
LIZARD POSE	217
YOGA FOR MEDITATION	**219**
THE ACCOMPLISHED POSE	219
AUSPICIOUS POSE	221
ANAL LOCK	223
YOGIC SLEEP	225
YOGA SEQUENCES FOR BEGINNERS	**227**
SUN SALUTATION	228
STANDING YOGA SEQUENCE	230
SEATED YOGA SEQUENCE	232
SUPINE SEQUENCE	235
BREATHING AND MEDITATION	**237**
BENEFITS OF PRANAYAMA	237
TYPES OF PRANAYAMA FOR BEGINNERS	239
PRACTICING PRANAYAMA AND MEDITATION	242
PARTING WORDS	**243**

Introduction

We thank you for downloading the book *Yoga for Beginners*, which is a well-planned guide to help beginners upgrade themselves to a healthy lifestyle.

This book gives an insight into the history of yoga and the benefits of practicing the ancient art. It's designed with a view to involving its readers in yogic practice for a better today and tomorrow.

The yoga poses included in the book are easy to do, not only for beginners but also for those with low flexibility levels. They were chosen taking into account factors including age, flexibility levels, and health conditions practitioners may be experiencing. Along with the images of the poses, you will find instructions on how to perform them. Regular practice of the yoga poses gives practitioners optimum benefits, both physically and psychologically.

The book helps you learn about

- the history of yoga
- the benefits of practicing yoga
- simple yoga poses for beginners with instructions and images
- yoga sequences
- yoga for specific health conditions
- avoiding mistakes
- dos and don'ts

We sincerely hope our book will help you begin to live a more healthy and balanced life. We wish you the very best in your yogic practice.

Thanks again for downloading the book.

What is Yoga?

Yoga, according to many from the West, consists of *asanas,* or postures. Yoga is considered in the West as one of the 'keep fit' exercises, and as an alternate therapy for physical conditions. Some practitioners choose yoga to build muscles. Many enrol in classes to find relief from stress. It is also believed by some in the West that yoga is a religion, and hence they equate practicing yoga to embracing the religion.

Is this really what yoga is all about? Does yoga in the East, in India, its native land, mean the same thing, and is it practiced by sages for similar purposes?

Is yoga an art? Does it represent a religion, or is it a religion in itself? Is yoga just another exercise to keep the body healthy?

Well then, what is yoga?

In truth, yoga is as much a religion as it is a physical exercise. It's not only a religion, and it could never be considered only an exercise. It's a balm and support to the spirit, as much as to the body.

Contrary to what is believed in the West, *asanas* (the poses) are not yoga, but only a part of it.

Yoga, which dates back thousands of years, is a body-mind practice. It is the union of your consciousness with supreme consciousness.

Yogis of the ancient days practiced and preached yoga not as a form of physical exercise, but as the path to unite body, mind, and soul, and achieve enlightenment. Mind modification is not emphasized in western yoga, but it is the purpose of the practice in the East. By modifying the mind, negative emotions are prevented, and the mind is tuned to meditate, to achieve self-realization.

Yoga co-ordinates the body and mind and elevates your spiritual state to where you may feel at one with universe. It helps you attain self-realization, a state in which ego is shed and your true self is realized. It is precisely this state which reveals your unlimited potential.

Yoga is a practice that promotes harmony within the self, and with the world. Since body and mind are interrelated, a health issue in your body will affect your mind, and stress in your mind will affect your health. For example, a headache may make you feel tired and irritated, and you may want to shut out the world. Likewise, stress may cause you to feel unwell and be short-tempered, and we know that chronic stress leads to various health conditions. Only if your body and mind are settled will you find peace within, and be in perfect harmony. Yoga helps you to achieve this state with *asanas* and *dhyana*.

Asanas, meaning postures, in yoga promote physical health. Asanas bring into action every part of your body from head to toe and hence performing them stimulates the function of organs.

Yoga is also one of the best practices to keep your mind healthy. While practicing yoga, your mind is naturally involved in what your body is doing, thereby improving your focus. While this directly helps your yogic practice, it also indirectly helps you by keeping your mind from wandering. Dhyana, meaning meditation, is a limb of yoga that promotes mental calm. The more the mind is at peace, better your mental health will be.

Yoga is unique because it co-ordinates body, mind, and soul. It not only calms the mind, but promotes spirituality. Spirituality is not about religion. It is a state of mind, a sense of being connected to the supreme consciousness, and it leads to self-realization. Yoga, thus, plays a great role in balancing your body, mind, and soul.

Yoga transcends race, religion, country, and every other boundary to benefit everyone. Simply put, yoga is a way of life.

Types of Yoga

There are many kinds of yoga, so a beginner might wonder what they are, and how to choose the best one for them. Below, we list some of the most common types, and talk a bit about them.

Ashtanga Yoga – Also known as Raja yoga and Eight Limbed yoga, Ashtanga yoga is the path of self-discipline. It is based on the philosophy of Yoga Sutra, authored by Sage Patanjali. He felt that there are eight stages to enlightenment, and each forms a limb in his philosophy. The eight limbs, or the eight practices, of Ashtanga yoga are as follows:

1) ***Yama*** – Meaning 'control,' yama refers to abiding by moral values such as not lying, not stealing, not being greedy, not being sensual, and not being violent. These are the 'don'ts' of Ashtanga yoga.

2) ***Niyama*** – Meaning 'non-control,' niyama refers to the 'dos' of yoga, which are developing personal qualities including cleanliness, contentment, austerity, introspection, and devotion.

3) ***Asana*** – refers to the practicing of yoga poses to promote physical and mental health.

4) ***Pranayama*** – performing breathing techniques for overall health

5) ***Pratyahara*** – Meaning 'withdrawal from the senses,' pratyahara serves as a transitional phase from previous limbs to subsequent limbs as the focus at this stage shifts from outward to inward, thereby promoting your yogic practice to higher levels.

6) **_Dharana_** – focusing on something specific, either internal or external, in order to clear and quiet the mind. Dharana prepares you for dhyana.

7) **_Dhyana_** – Unlike in dharana, in dhyana you are in absolute reality where you are totally aware and present in the moment. Attaining the state requires consistent practice.

8) **_Samadhi_** – You experience a tranquil state in which you remain aware of truth.

Hatha Yoga – 'Ha' in Hatha means 'sun,' which refers to the right side of the body, and 'tha' means 'moon,' referring to the left side. Hatha yoga involves practicing asanas and pranayama to balance both sides. Hatha yoga practice improves your fitness levels.

Kundalini Yoga – Also known as Laya yoga, Kundalini yoga awakens Kundalini, the life force, which is located at the base of spine. Kundalini yoga connects the seven chakras, the body's energy centers, and helps to achieve inner peace.

Mantra Yoga – Mantra yoga is a practice in which mantras are chanted rhythmically. Mantra chanting improves focus while meditating. Mantra yoga practice elevates your level of consciousness.

A Brief History of Yoga

Yoga, originating in India and now practiced throughout the world, is a very ancient science of body, mind, and soul. According to references in ancient scripts, yoga originated over five thousand years ago. Just how long before that is a question that will likely remain unanswered.

A common explanation of where the name 'yoga' came from is that it is derived from Yuj, a Sanskrit word meaning 'union.' However, because it is so old, we'll never know for sure.

What we do know is that even before the times when written records mentioned yoga, the practice existed. From gurus to disciples, and from stone carvings to palm leaf manuscripts, the teachings of yoga spread. *Rig Veda*, a collection of ancient Sanskrit hymns, is believed to be from the Vedic period, between 1500 BCE to 500 BCE. It mentions yoga. However, the origin of yoga cannot be assigned to this period, as *Rig Veda* was codified around this period, but we know it was handed down to successive generations by word of mouth much earlier than that.

An ancient writer, Sage Patanjali, compiled *Yoga Sutras* in which he explains the essence of yoga in scientific terms. He says yoga has the ability to control fluctuations of the mind. He describes Ashtanga yoga, the Eight Limbed practice, which includes adhering to moral values, performing asanas, pranayama, and meditating so as to reach the ultimate goal – enlightenment that leads to liberation.

Based on the available history of yoga, we see some evolution of the practice. During the Vedic times, yoga practice was more oriented towards moral values and spiritual life. The three basic

Vedic yoga types are Mantra yoga, Prana yoga, and Dhyana Yoga.

Following that, in pre-classical times, meditation and knowing one's inner self were the main focus of yoga practice.

The classical period was an important one in the history of yoga. It is during this period that Sage Patanjali compiled *Yoga Sutras*, the authoritative work on yoga. Classical yoga is based on Ashtanga yoga, the Eight Limbed practice.

Post-classical yoga teaches us to live in the present and learn acceptance. This time period saw a shift in focus, from liberation to healing and healthy living. This period established a strong foundation for Hatha yoga practice.

Throughout all these periods the essence of yoga has been the same, only how it was applied differed.

The Philosophy Behind Yoga

The main philosophy of yoga is to steady the mind so that peace, self-realization, and enlightenment can be achieved.

Yoga philosophy is about guiding you to reach spiritual heights, which is what life should be all about. Being materialistic lets you enjoy some pleasures, but to enjoy the essence of life, your mind should be spiritually oriented. According to the philosophy of yoga, being materialistic, giving in to sensory pleasures, not following moral codes, lacking in good physical and mental health, and emotional blocks such as anger, envy, and stress come in the way of spiritual progress.

To achieve peace of mind and progress towards enlightenment, asanas and breathing techniques should be followed. Yoga philosophy recommends the Eight Limbed practice, which as we've seen, involves following moral codes, and being pure in thought and action. It means practicing yoga postures and breathing techniques, and meditating, so your mind is liberated and the moment of self-realization is achieved.

Ashtanga yoga, Hatha yoga, Kundalini yoga, and Mantra yoga are the types of yoga that involve these practices for optimum health.

The Health Benefits of Yoga

The benefits of yoga are numerous. That yoga has been practiced since ancient times is proof of how well yoga works for the body, mind, and soul. The poses involve stretching in all directions, bending backwards and forwards, and twisting – all of which work the entire body. Yoga poses stimulate organs and glands and optimize their performance.

Practicing of yoga regularly helps to keep you strong both physically and mentally. Here is a list of important benefits of yoga.

1) Overall support for the body
Practicing yoga benefits your whole body. Yoga oxygenates the body, improves blood circulation, promotes physical fitness, and supports overall health.

2) Boosts lung function
Yoga expands the chest, strengthens the respiratory muscles, and relieves airway obstruction, thereby improving respiratory function and aiding in curing respiratory conditions, including asthma and bronchitis.

3) Protects heart health
Yoga supports heart health. It maintains healthy blood pressure levels and lowers bad cholesterol. As it helps with weight loss, it reduces the risk of heart conditions. Yoga also relieves stress, one of the most common causes for heart-related issues, thereby protecting the heart.

4) Improves digestive function
Many people don't realize that poor digestion is the root cause of many illnesses. Improper digestion causes stomach disorders, headaches, and various other health issues. Yoga strengthens

digestive function and reduces the risks of other health conditions. It also increases awareness of the body, which may help to reveal problematic foods, and aid in better food choices being made overall.

5) Boosts immunity
Yoga supports the functions of all systems of the body, and thereby promotes immunity. The stronger you get, the more your body is able to fight off pathogens and infection.

6) Strengthens the nervous system
The twisting of the body and holding of certain yoga asanas strengthens the spine and supports spine health. Restorative yoga poses and breathing techniques stimulate the parasympathetic nervous system. Also, by improving the body's ability to handle stress, yoga regulates nervous system.

7) Strengthens muscular system
Yoga tones, contracts, and strengthens the muscles. It involves every muscle in your body. The involuntary muscles, such as heart muscles, are controlled by the autonomic nervous system, which is strengthened by yoga poses. Balancing yoga poses strengthen muscles and improve resistance.

8) Improves flexibility
Yoga improves your range of motion by increasing your flexibility levels. Stretching, twisting, lengthening, and contracting involved in your yogic practice increase your flexibility to amazing levels. Every joint and muscle gets its share of movement while you practice yoga, and hence stiffness in joints is prevented.

Additionally, when we improve strength and flexibility, we get better balance. This will help to reduce falls and the associated injuries.

9) Aids weight loss

One of the most common reasons given by practitioners to begin yoga is to achieve weight loss goals. Obesity is a great cause of concern as it foretells many health hazards including diabetes and heart conditions. Regular practice of yoga reduces excess fat and body weight by maintaining a healthy metabolism.

10) Relieves pain

Studies show that yoga reduces pain perception. It improves the function of organs and glands, thereby relieving and minimizing the occurrence of pain. If you have frequent headaches due to indigestion, practicing yoga will help you as it will strengthen the digestive system.

Yoga is also effective in curing muscular cramps, thereby relieving pain associated with those.

11) Postpones aging

A compelling reason to practice yoga is its anti-aging effects. Yoga improves blood circulation, and hence your body gets more of the oxygen and nutrients it needs to keep you looking young. By energizing your body, yoga makes you feel much younger. It improves your flexibility, which normally reduces as you age. Also, by improving your strength, balance, and flexibility, yoga keeps you agile. Regular practice of yoga helps you stay constantly aware of your body, making you more likely to avoid foods and other habits that may not be good for you. It also corrects your posture, which reduces discomfort and helps to postpone symptoms of old age.

12) Relieves PMS and menopausal symptoms

Yoga relieves pre-menstrual syndrome and menopause symptoms such as headache, abdominal pain, nausea, cramps, bloating, and back pain. It soothes the nerves and has a calming effect to relieve you of stress and mood swings that are normally present during the menstrual cycle. By practicing yoga regularly, these symptoms can be drastically reduced, or even prevented.

13) Relieves stress
Stress can trigger various health conditions. Chronic stress can cause headaches, hyperacidity in the stomach, and can affect your blood pressure and blood sugar levels. Physical workouts generally work as stress reliever. Yoga doubles that effect, as it works at psychological level as well as a physical one. It helps you to achieve a balanced state of mind. Pranayama, yogic breathing techniques, relax your mind, energize your body and relieve stress.

14) Spiritual benefits
The essence of yoga is spirituality. Asanas, breathing techniques, and meditation lead you in a spiritual path. You let go of control, release the ego, and become aware of your inner self. You will be in perfect harmony with the world. Your mind is purified, and your outlook on life is positive.

Yoga can also

- balance hormones and cure hormone disorders, including those of the thyroid
- help cure vision problems such as long- and short-sightedness, through certain eye exercises
- relieve arthritic conditions
- improve athletic performance
- cure insomnia
- detoxify the body
- promote blood flow to the reproductive organs, and aid in fertility
- boost memory power
- improve focus
- promote self-confidence
- cure, or relieve the symptoms of depression

100 Yoga Poses for Beginners

Your reason for rolling out the yoga mat can be to achieve fitness goals, or relieve a health condition, or to advance spiritually. To fulfill your aim, you need to start with beginner poses. These poses prepare your body to progress to advanced yoga poses.

Given below are one hundred yoga poses for beginners. The first chapter covers the most common basic poses that a beginner can start with to adapt their body and mind to yoga culture. The above-mentioned chapter is followed by poses that are classified into appropriate sections to enable you to choose the required topic or area of focus with ease.

It's great if you are able to do these poses perfectly in the first few attempts, but if you find some (or many) of the poses tough, never push yourself too hard. It just takes some time and repetition. With practice, you will comfortably master the poses.

To assist further in your progress, we have added a few intermediate poses under each category. Once you are comfortable with the poses for beginners, you may try the intermediate poses. Again, this is only a beginning.

*Important Note: There are health conditions and ailments that can be aggravated by some yoga poses – for instance, some stretches should be avoided if you're pregnant, nursing or have sustained injuries recently or in the past. Please consult your doctor if you have any questions about whether yoga is safe for you, or whether any restrictions should be observed.

Guidelines for Yoga Practice

Here are the general guidelines for practicing yoga.

- Emptying the bladder before practice is highly recommended. However, not having bowel movements should not stop you from practicing.
- Keep the surrounding area clean. It is not only healthy, but also serves as an inspiration to the mind and spirit.
- With the exception of thunderbolt pose, all other yoga poses should be practiced only on an empty stomach. Drinking a glass of water before practice is allowed. After completing your yoga practice, wait for at least 20 minutes to drink or eat.
- Those who can perform the poses only in the evening should do so four hours after having your meal.
- Performing yoga after a bath is fine, but if you start your day with yoga, you need to wait for 30 minutes afterward to have a bath.
- Perform yoga in a properly ventilated space.
- Practice yoga on a mat or a folded blanket.
- Wear clothes that you are comfortable with and that support movement.
- Avoid distractions of all sorts.
- Never push yourself hard to accomplish a pose.
- Avoid practicing yoga when you are experiencing illness, after a long journey, or when you feel exhausted.
- Your goal for practicing yoga can be anything from meeting fitness goals, to weight loss, or improving a health condition. Determine your goal and work out a practice that best suits you. Include the type of asanas that support your goal. Include variations. Instead of practicing same poses every day, practice different sets of poses that help you achieve your goals.
- Pay attention to how you breathe. Coordinating your breath with practice produces optimum results. Focusing on breathing also keeps your mind focused in your practice.

Basic Yoga Poses

Let's start at the beginning. Given below are simple, basic yoga poses that tone your body and prepare you for a wonderful yoga session. Practicing these poses regularly not only improves your flexibility, but also promotes overall health.

Staff Pose

Staff pose, or staff posture, is the basic pose for all seated poses. All seated poses begin here, so be sure you are comfortable with it before you move on.

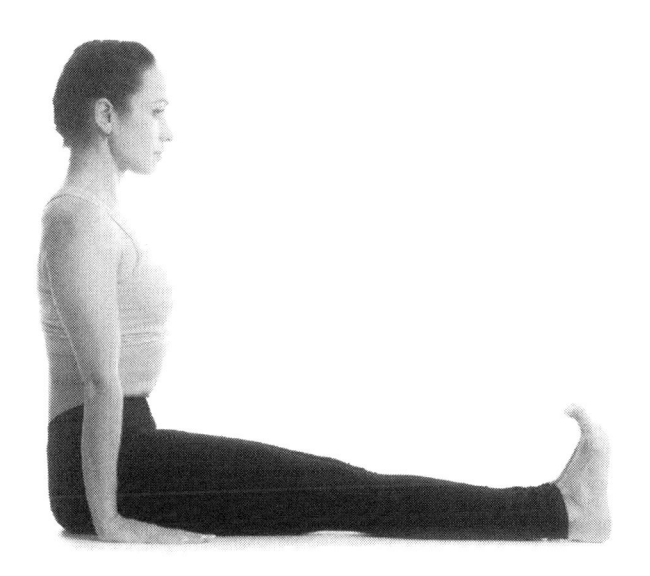

Instructions
1. Sit down with your legs stretched forward. Keep your hands by your sides.
2. Keep your sit bones firmly on the ground.
3. Press your heels firmly on the ground so that your weight is evenly distributed along your legs.

4. Engage the thigh muscles and keep the thighs firmly to the ground.
5. Place the palms by the sides of your hips. Keep your fingertips pointed forward.
6. Placing the hands firmly on the floor, and lengthen your spine. Lift your torso so that the pelvis is slightly forward.
7. Keep your feet straight, toes pointing upward.
8. Expand your shoulders and keep your chest lifted.
9. Gently pull your belly button in.
10. Lift your chin so that your crown is pointed towards the ceiling.
11. Look straight ahead.
12. Remain in the pose for one minute.

Benefits

- Stretches and strengthens the spine, shoulders, and abdomen
- Stretches the back
- Reduces symptoms of asthma
- Strengthens the hips
- Relieves sciatic pain
- Improves awareness of your posture, and so helps you to correct it
- Increases core strength
- Improves focus
- Relieves stress

Note

If your lower back strains, sit on a folded blanket so your hips are elevated, thereby reducing the pressure on your lower back. You can use a wall for support, so that you can correct your posture, as sitting against the wall makes you aware of your body's shape.

Caution

Avoid practicing the pose if you have injured your wrists or lower back.

Half Lotus Pose

Half lotus pose is a simpler version of lotus pose, which is considered the best pose for meditation. Practicing half lotus pose will help you perform lotus pose with ease.

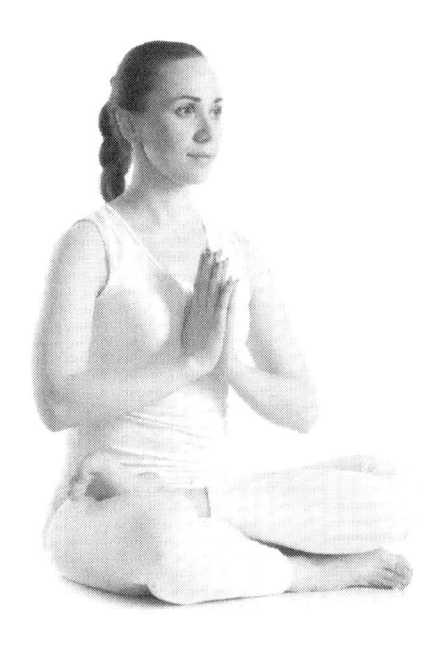

Instructions
1. Sit in staff pose.
2. Bend your right leg and place your right foot on the left thigh. The right foot should be at the uppermost part of the thigh so that your right heel touches the abdomen.
3. Slide your left foot under the right thigh.
4. Let the palms be on your thighs in chin mudra, in which you bring the tips of your thumb and index finger together in light contact and the other three fingers stretched.
5. Straighten your spine.
6. Keep your eyes closed.
7. Remain in the pose for one minute.

Benefits
- Stretches and strengthens the spine and back
- Stretches the hips and legs
- Promotes blood flow to the pelvic region
- Relieves menstrual pain
- Relieves stress
- Cures mild depression
- Promotes calm

Caution
Those with severe hip or knee problems should perform this pose with caution.

Seated Mountain Pose

Seated mountain pose improves spine alignment, which helps beginners to correct their posture.

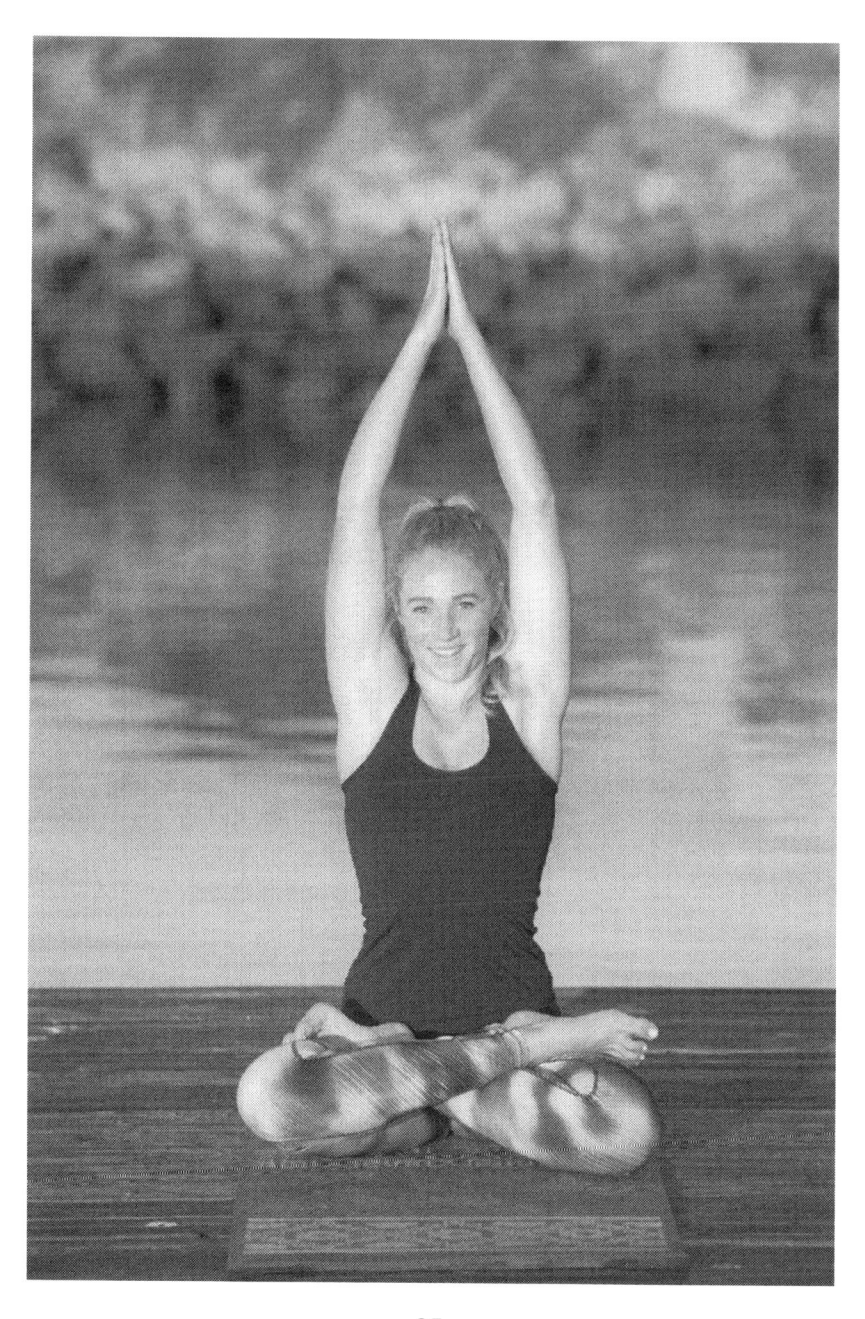

Instructions
1. Sit in the posture that is most comfortable to you, though being seated in lotus pose is ideal. However, you can sit in half lotus pose or easy pose (legs crossed normally, feet tucked under the thighs).
2. Inhale. Stretch your hands sideways, keeping the palms facing downwards.
3. Exhale as you lift your hands over your head.
4. Bring the hands together.
5. Keep your elbows straight.
6. Lengthen your spine and lift the hands straight.
7. Remain in the pose for 30 seconds.
8. Come out of the pose by releasing the finger lock and lowering your hands to the thighs.

Benefits
- Aligns the spine
- Tones the back and relieves back pain
- Stretches the shoulders and relieves shoulder pain
- Calms the mind

Note
Those with knee injuries or who cannot sit on the floor with the legs crossed can perform this pose sitting on a chair.

Hero Pose

Hero pose can be a bit challenging for a beginner, but this is one pose that you need to master to make you more flexible and ready for tougher poses.

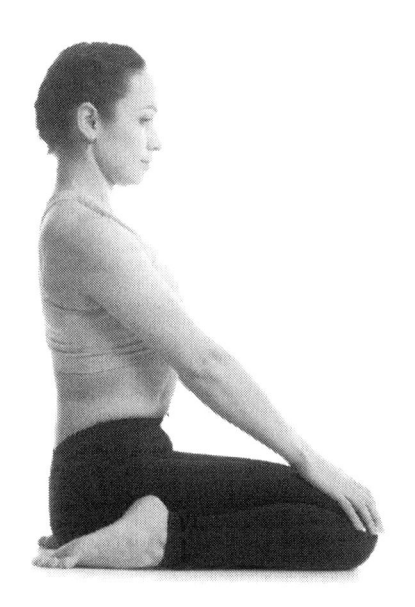

Instructions
1. Kneel on the mat.
2. Keep your thighs together and place your feet hip-width apart. The tops of your feet should be on the floor.
3. Exhale and sit on the space between your feet.
4. Your lower legs should be on the outer sides of your thighs.
5. Turn the thighs inward.
6. Pull your spine up.
7. Lift your hands sideways and up. Lock the fingers and turn your palms upwards. Alternatively, the hands may be placed on the knees.
8. Keep your eyes closed, or fix your gaze straight ahead.

9. Remain in the pose for one minute. On getting comfortable with the pose, you can increase the duration up to 5 minutes.
10. To come out of the pose, place your hands on the floor by your sides. Lift your butt slightly and cross your ankles so that you can sit back on the floor. Now stretch your legs forward.

Benefits
- Stretches the hips, thighs, knees, ankles, and feet
- Tones thigh muscles
- Improves digestion
- Relieves gas
- Relieves symptoms of asthma
- Relieves menopausal symptoms
- Improves flat foot if done from an early age
- Improves posture

Note
If sitting down between the legs hurts your ankles, you may place a block between your feet and sit on it.

Caution
Those with knee or ankle injuries should avoid practicing this pose. Also, hero pose should not be practiced by those with heart problems.

Half Squat Pose

Half squat pose is an excellent pose for beginners to practice stretching and making the hips and legs flexible. It is one of the best beginner poses for the lower body.

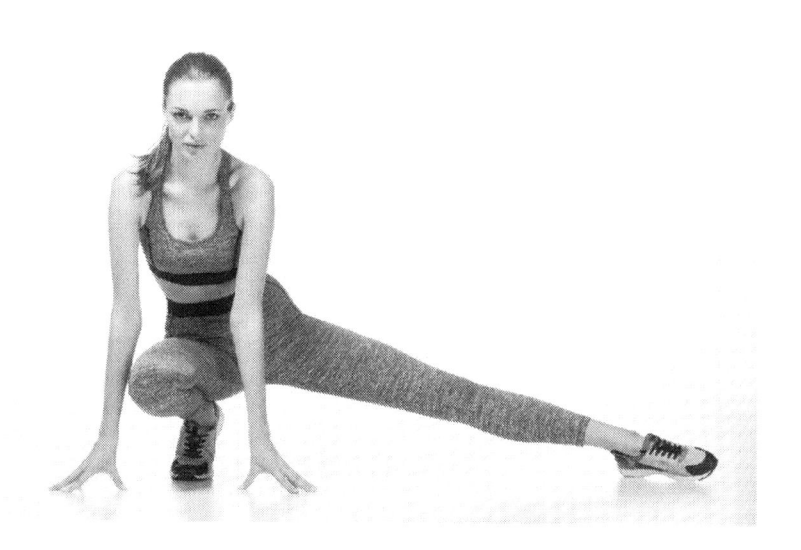

Instructions
1. Go on all fours with your wrists in line with your shoulders, and knees aligned with your hips.
2. Walk your hands towards your feet.
3. As your hands get closer, lean back to place your feet flat on the floor. Now your hips will be down, but not touching the ground.
4. Place your palms in front of you on the floor.
5. With palms firmly to the ground, stretch your right leg to your right.
6. Stretch your right leg as much as possible. The further you stretch, the closer your hip will get to your left heel.
7. Hold the pose for 30 seconds.

8. Come out of the pose by bringing your extended leg back into a squat.
9. Repeat the same with the other leg.

Benefits
- Opens and strengthens the hips
- Stretches and strengthens the legs
- Improves flexibility of the knees
- Boosts metabolism
- Tones abdominal muscles
- Improves digestion
- Promotes balance and stability

Note
If you find balancing difficult, you can place your palms on the floor or a block, instead of keeping your palms together in front of your chest.

Caution
Avoid practicing the pose if you have a knee or foot injury. Do not practice the pose during menstruation.

Tiger Pose

Tiger pose is not fierce, as the name sounds. It is one of the beginner poses that promotes flexibility.

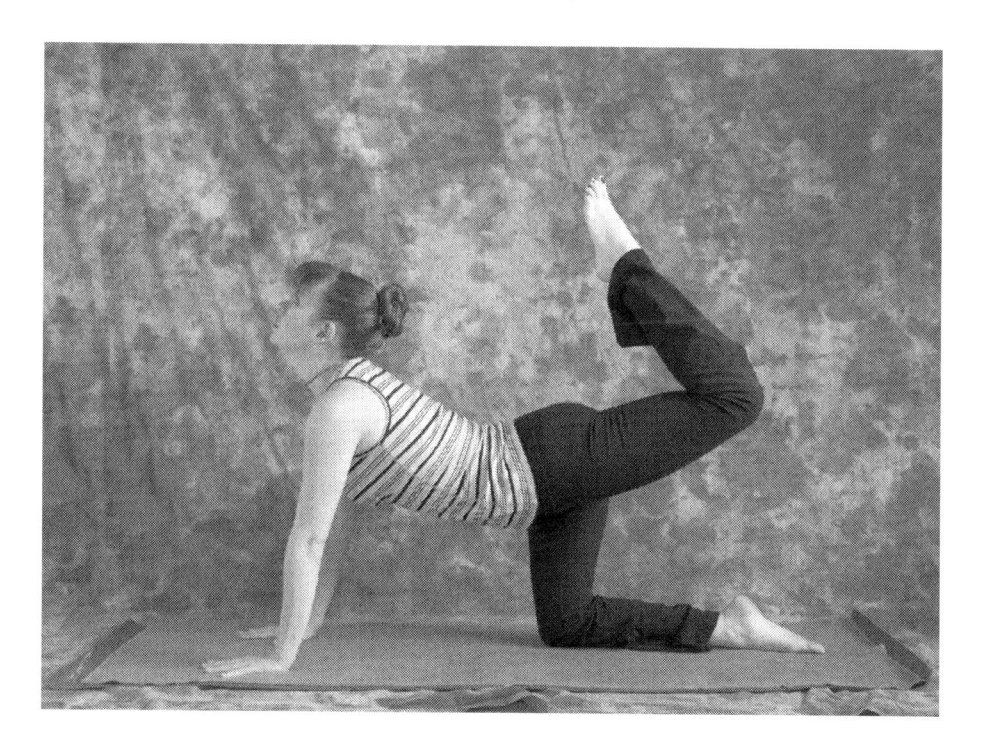

Instructions

1. Go on all fours with your palms and knees on the ground. Keep your wrists aligned with your shoulders and your knees to your hips.
2. Exhale. Draw your right knee in towards your face. Lower your head to bring the forehead and knee into contact.
3. Inhale as you bring the right leg out of contact with your forehead, and extend the leg back without straightening the knee, so your right foot is angled towards your head. While your right leg is extended, the right pelvis should remain in place.
4. Lift your head to look up, stretching the neck as much as possible.

5. Repeat the movement up to 8 times.
6. After 8 repetitions, place your right knee on the floor.
7. Repeat the same steps with your left knee.
8. Do 3 to 5 rounds.

Benefits
- Stretches the spine
- Tones the back muscles
- Strengthens the core
- Strengthens the shoulders, arms, wrists, and legs
- Tones and strengthens the abdominal muscles and hips
- Reduces sciatic pain
- Boosts blood circulation
- Stimulates the nervous system and reproductive system
- Improves digestion
- Reduces excess fat in hips and thighs

Note
Place a folded blanket under your knees in case of discomfort. If your neck hurts, keep your head and neck parallel with the floor.

Caution
If you have severe wrists, hip, or knee injuries, you should avoid this pose.

One Handed Tiger Pose

One handed tiger pose is a variation of tiger pose. It gives depth to your yoga practice.

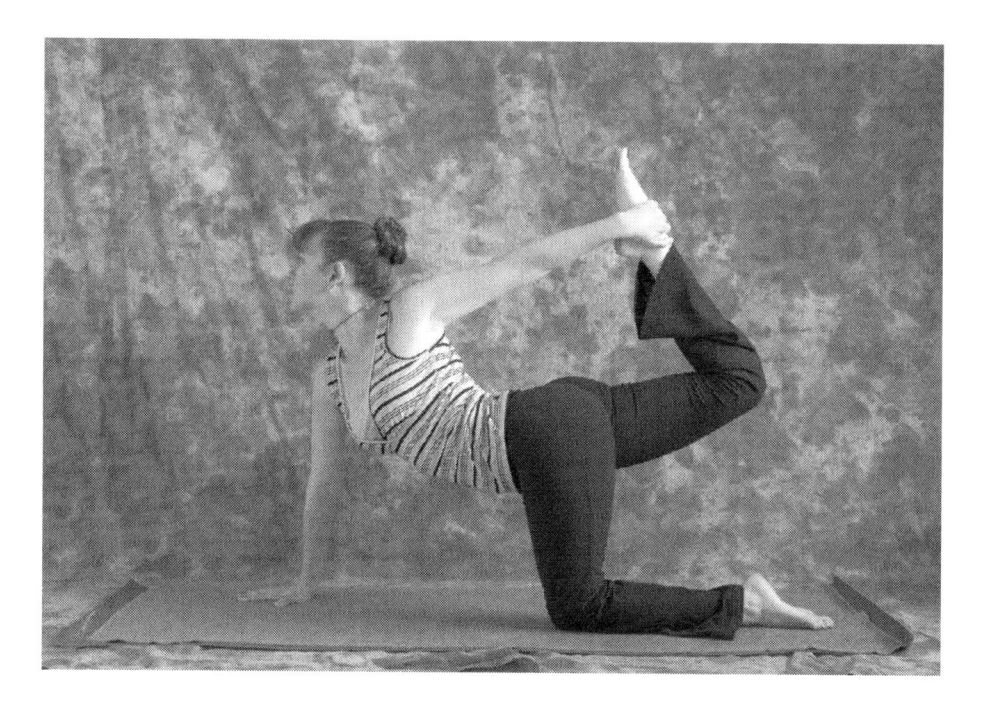

Instructions
1. Go on all fours. Lift your right foot up. The right knee should be bent.
2. Gently arch your spine.
3. Lift the left hand, shifting your weight to the right hand.
4. Stretch your left hand behind you, to hold the inside of the right ankle.
5. Supported by your hand, lift the right leg higher.
6. Raise your head and look forward.
7. Remain in the pose for 30 seconds.
8. Repeat the same steps with the other hand and leg.

Benefits
- Stretches the arms, shoulders, back, and legs
- Boosts energy
- Stimulates abdominal organs

Note
Place a folded blanket under the knees in case of discomfort.

Caution
Avoid practicing this pose if you have chronic injury in your shoulders, arms, hips, or legs.

Lion Pose

Lion pose promotes flexibility of the legs and ankles, and hence it is one of those ideal poses for beginners. The pose is considered to be the eradicator of diseases.

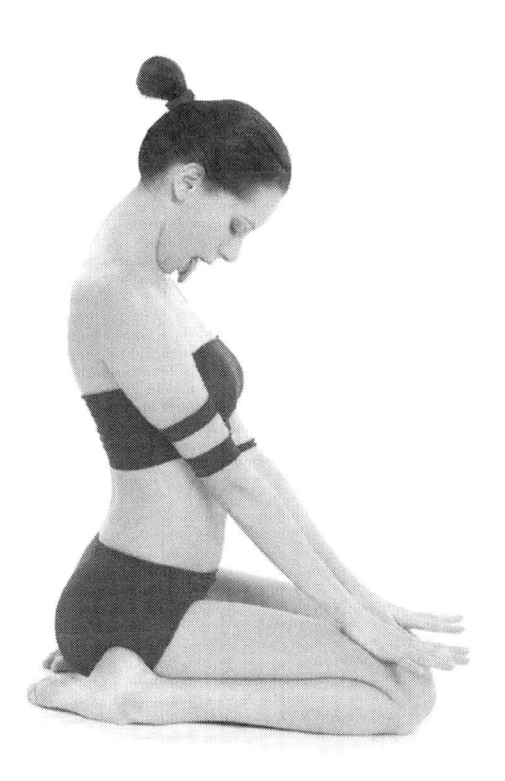

Instructions
1. Kneel down on the floor.
2. Sit down on your heels, bending the knees. Move the knees apart so there is space between your thighs. Lower your body down between the thighs.
3. Place your palms down on the thighs just before the knees. Spread the fingers out.

4. Open your mouth and bring the tongue out. Stretch the tongue out and down as much as possible.
5. Fix your gaze between the eyebrows as best you can. Keep the eyes open. You can also look at the tip of your nose.
6. Inhale and exhale. While exhaling, make a sound to imitate a lion's breathing. However, you can also breathe normally.
7. Remain in the pose until you feel comfortable.

Benefits
- Improves voice quality and helps with stuttering
- Cures defects in the nose, mouth, and ears
- Stimulates the nerves of the eyes
- Cures bad breath
- Relieves throat infection
- Relaxes the facial muscles, removes wrinkles, and promotes a youthful appearance
- Improves the function of the respiratory system
- Tones the abdomen
- Relieves stress

Bound Angle Pose

Balancing bound angle pose is a basic balancing posture which is ideal for beginners.

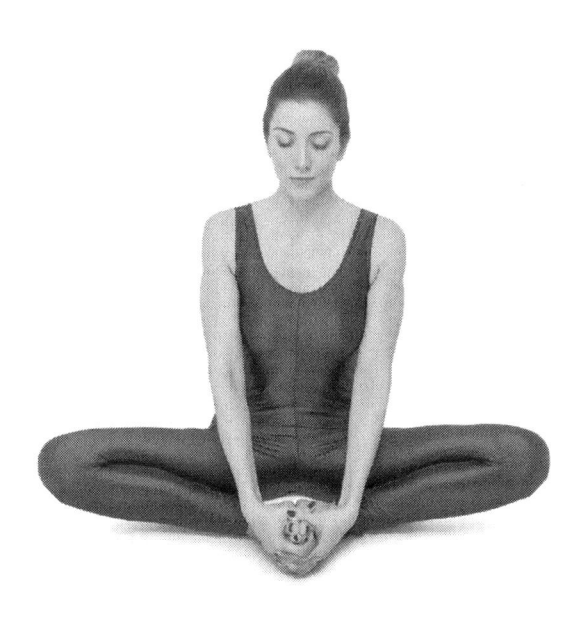

Instructions
1. Start in staff pose (p19), in which you sit on the floor with your legs stretched out in front of you.
2. Bend your legs and place the soles of the feet against each other.
3. Wrap your fingers around the toes.
4. Relax and push your shoulders back, so the chest is pressed forward.
5. Inhale and exhale slowly. Maintain the pose for 1 to 2 minutes

Variation Balancing *Bound Angle Pose*

1. Inhale and lean back and lift the feet off the floor.
2. Gradually lift the feet further up until they are in line with heart.
3. Bring the chest and feet closer.
4. Remain in the pose for 30 seconds.
5. To come out of the pose, place your feet on the floor while exhaling.

Benefits
- Opens the hips
- Tones the abdomen and back
- Strengthens the upper body
- Improves focus
- Promotes creativity
- Boosts self-confidence
- Improves balance

Caution
Avoid practicing this pose if you have any injury in your arms, shoulders, hips, or knees.

One Legged Boat Pose

One legged boat pose prepares you for boat pose and its advanced variation.

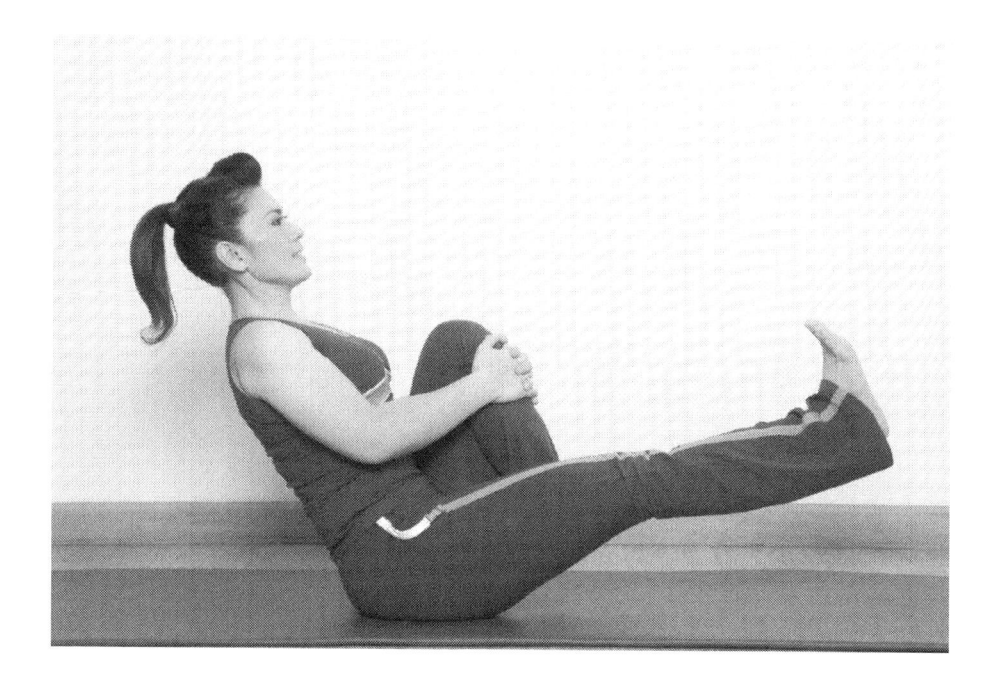

Instructions
1. Sit in staff pose (p19), in which you sit on the floor extending your feet in front of you.
2. Bend the left foot towards the right thigh.
3. Stretch your arms over the extended leg, keeping them parallel to the ground. Your palms should face each other.
4. With inhalation, lean back and lift your right leg up.
5. Relax your shoulders, and lift your chest.
6. Remain in the pose for 30 seconds.
7. Repeat the same process using the other leg.

Benefits
- Strengthens the core muscles
- Tones the back
- Stretches the legs
- Improves balance

Note
If balancing in this pose is difficult, hold the foot using a yoga strap.

Caution
Those with any injury to the neck, shoulders, hips, or knees should not perform this pose.

Wide Angle Seated Forward Bend

The Wide Angle Seated Forward Bend is a leg stretch pose for beginners. The pose introduces you to a leg stretch that opens the hips and is a good to warm-up for the entire legs and hips. It will prepare you for twisting poses, wide-legs standing poses and some seated poses.

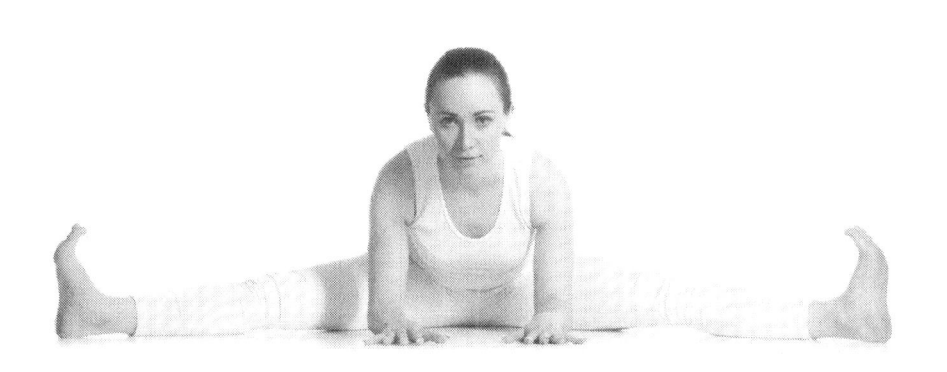

Instructions

1. From the staff pose (p19), lean your torso back slightly on your hands.
2. Lift and open your legs into a 90° angle.
3. Push your hands into the floor and then slide your buttocks forward to widen your legs more.
4. Turn your thighs outward and pin your outer thighs into the floor, pointing your kneecaps toward the ceiling. Stretch your soles through your heels toward your body.

5. Walk your hands forward between your legs, keeping your arms long as you do. Emphasize moving from the hip joints rather than the waist, and keep lengthening your front torso. If you start bending from the waist, stop and start lengthening from your pubis to your navel, continuing forward as far as possible.
6. Ideally, increase the bend after each exhalation until you feel comfortably stretched in the back of your legs. Hold the pose for a minute or longer.

Benefits
- Stretches and strengthens the spine, hips, and legs
- Improves the function of abdominal organs
- Relieves stress
- Promotes focus

Caution
Avoid practicing this pose if you have health conditions such as injury to your back, hips, or knees. Do not practice the pose if you have a headache.

Half Bow Pose

Half bow pose is a back-bending yoga pose that is done lying on the stomach. It shows beginners an effective way to improve flexibility.

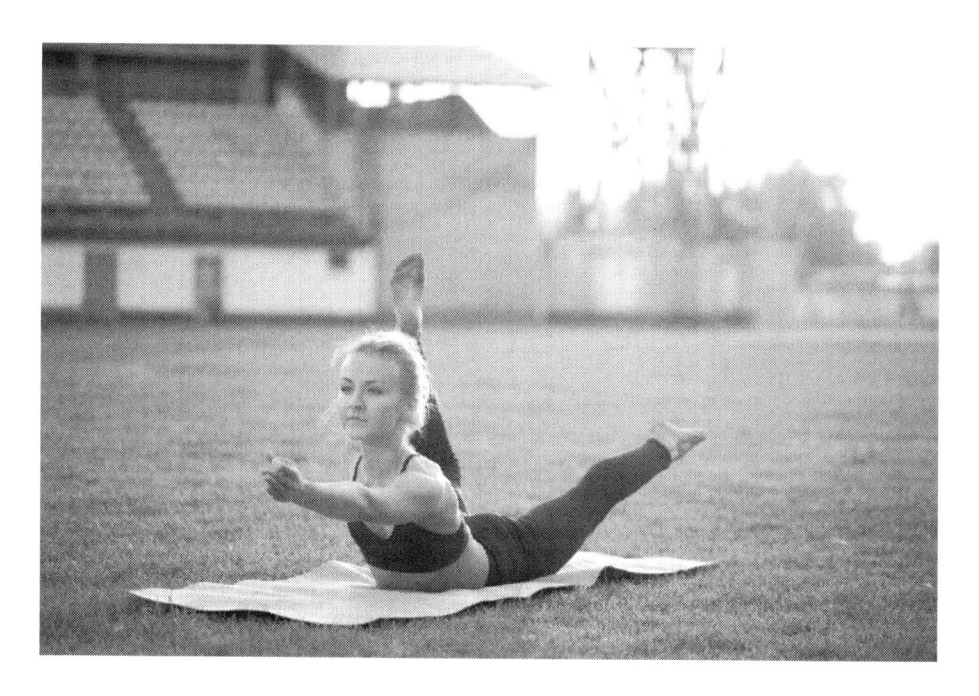

Instructions
1. Lie on your stomach, keeping your legs stretched out straight and your hands by your sides. Place your chin on the floor.
2. Stretch your right arm out in front of you. Keep your palm facing down.
3. Bend your right knee.
4. Stretch your left hand behind your back and hold the ankle of the right leg.
5. Inhale as you lift your head and chest off the floor. Simultaneously, lift the right thigh, supported by your left hand. Lift the leg high.
6. Lift your left hand off the floor and stretch it out straight.

7. Remain in the pose for 30 seconds.
8. Repeat the same steps with the other leg and hand.

Benefits
- Stretches the spine and improves its flexibility
- Tones the back muscles
- Strengthens the hips
- Stretches the shoulders, arms, and legs
- Strengthens the respiratory system and relieves respiratory disorders, including asthma
- Stimulates the abdominal organs and boosts the function of the liver, kidneys, and reproductive system
- Energizes the whole body
- Improves balance

Note
If you have difficulty reaching your ankle, loop a yoga strap around your foot and hold it with your hand. You may keep your extended hand on the ground if lifting it is difficult.

Caution
Those with any injury to the neck, shoulders, arms, hips, or legs should avoid practicing this pose.

Crocodile Pose

Crocodile pose is a resting pose that offers its share of benefits. It is among the easiest poses for beginners, and a rewarding one too, for the efforts taken on the mat.

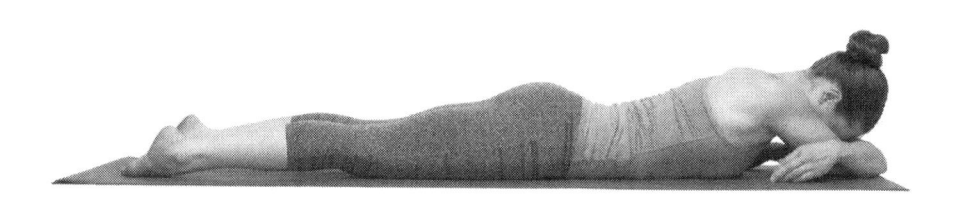

Instructions
1. Lie down on the yoga mat on your stomach.
2. The second step has several variations. You can fold your arms and place your head on them, or you can place your elbows on the ground, lift your forearms and hold your chin in your palms. You can also place your palms on the opposite shoulders with your elbows touching the ground and your forehead on one of your forearms.
3. Keep your legs stretched out and separated.
4. Remain in the pose until you are comfortable, or until you are ready to perform another pose.

Benefits
- Relaxes your body and mind
- Relieves fatigue
- Relaxes the spine and shoulders
- Lowers high blood pressure
- Improves heart health
- Cures back pain
- Relieves physical and psychological stress

Thread the Needle Pose

Thread the needle pose helps with conscious breathing. Breathing the correct way is an internal part of yogic practice. Thread the needle pose helps you achieve focus in your breathing.

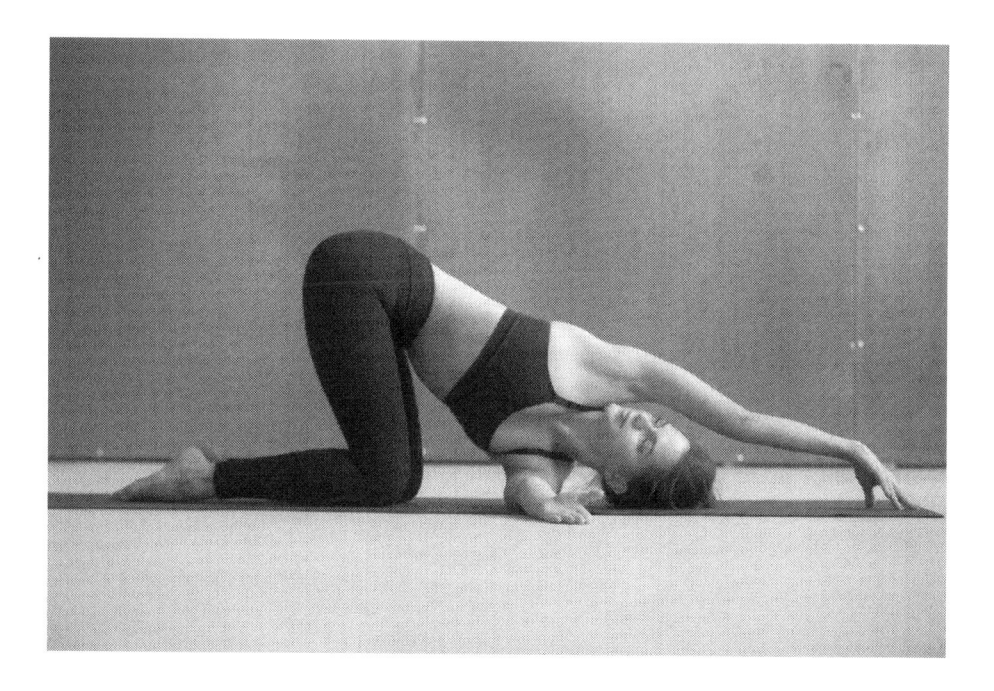

Instructions
1. Go on all fours, aligning your wrists with your shoulders and your knees with your hips.
2. Tuck in your toes so they point forward.
3. Inhale as you lift your right hand off the floor.
4. Stretch your right hand to the left side, under your torso and between the arm and leg. Simultaneously, lower the right side of your head to the floor.
5. Stretch your right arm further to your left. This will cause your torso to twist. Keep the palm facing upward.
6. Remain in the pose for 30 seconds.
7. Repeat the same steps on the other side.

Benefits
- Opens the shoulders
- Stretches the shoulders, arms, and hips
- Promotes blood flow to the upper extremities
- Improves the function of abdominal organs
- Improves digestion
- Aids in detoxification
- Relieves stress
- Promotes calm

Note
Place a folded blanket under your knees if they hurt.

Caution
Those with high or low blood pressure, heart conditions, or any injuries to the neck, shoulders, back, or hips should not practice this pose. Do not practice the pose if you have a headache.

Eye of the Needle Pose

Eye of the needle pose makes the hips flexible, and hence is recommended for beginners. Tight hips are a common problem, usually owing to lifestyle.

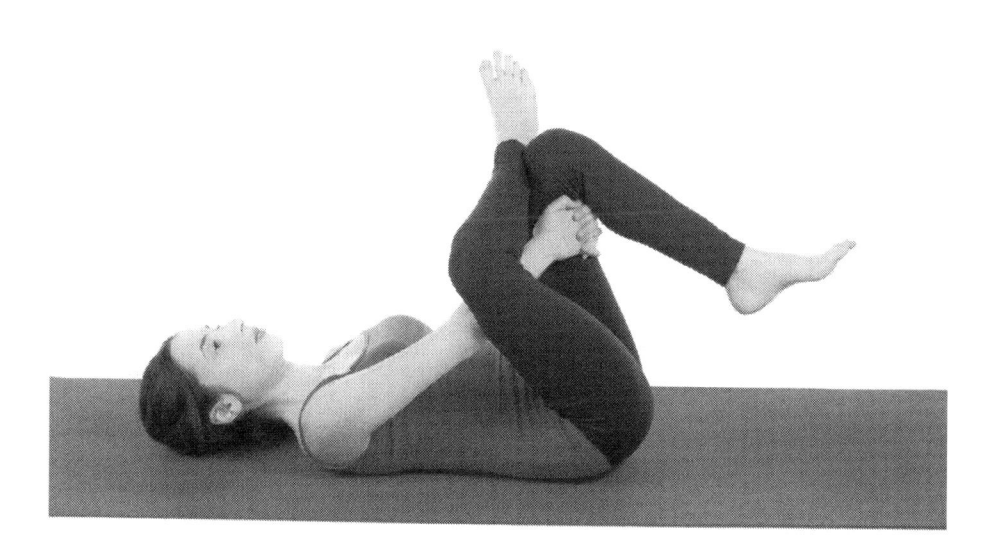

Instructions
1. Lie down on your back. Bend your knees and keep the soles of your feet on the floor.
2. Place the right ankle on the outer side of the left thigh. The right knee should be angled away from your torso.
3. Pull your left foot toward your body, and slide your right hand through the legs and curl it around the left thigh. You can also clasp your left thigh with your hands.
4. Pressing with your hands, draw the left thigh closer to your chest.
5. Relax the feet.
6. Remain in the pose for 30 seconds.
7. Repeat the same process on the other side.

Benefits
- Stretches the hips
- Increases leg flexibility
- Prepares the body for poses that require higher flexibility levels
- Promotes calm

Caution
Avoid practicing the pose if you have a knee injury.

Happy Baby Pose

Happy baby pose is yet another perfect pose for tight hips and to relax the lower back.

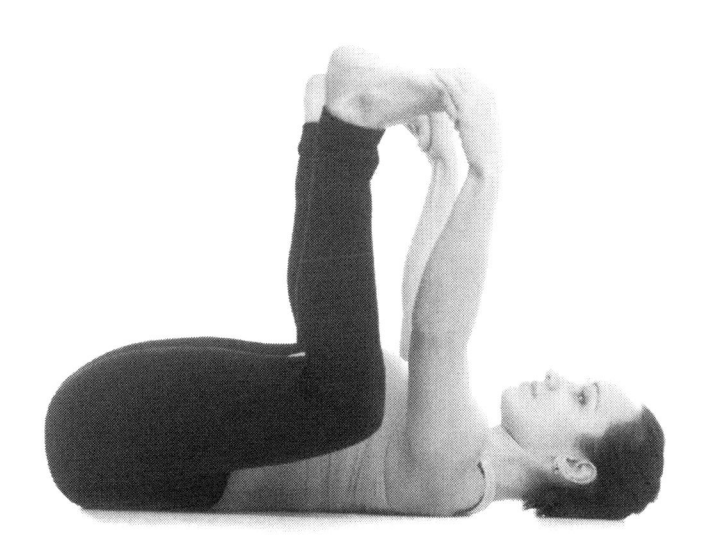

Instructions
1. Lie on your back, stretching your legs straight and keeping your hands by your sides.
2. Exhale as you bend your knees towards your belly. Inhale.
3. Exhale as you stretch your hands to hold your feet, gripping the outer sides.
4. Your ankles should be positioned above your knees, and your thighs should be over the abdomen.
5. Place your tailbone on the mat and release the pelvis by stretching your spine. Your hips should be on the mat.
6. Hold on to the pose for one minute.
7. Exhale and release your legs to the mat to come out of the pose.

Benefits
- Opens the chest and hips
- Stretches the shoulders
- Strengthens the biceps
- Stretches the spine and tones the back
- Tones the abdominal muscles
- Stretches the inner thighs
- Relieves fatigue
- Promotes calm

Note
Those who are unable to reach their feet can use yoga strap to wrap the feet and hold the ends of the strap. If you have neck pain, you can use a thick blanket folded under the head.

Caution
Practice this pose with caution in case of injury to the hips, knees, and ankles.

Mountain Pose

Mountain pose is the foundation of all standing poses. Seemingly simple, the pose requires you to stay focused on your body and its alignment.

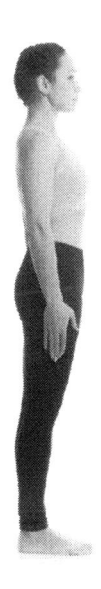

Instructions
1. Stand straight with your feet placed together. Your weight should be evenly distributed across the four corners of your feet. Keep your arms by your sides.
2. Lift your toes and release them to the mat one at a time.
3. Relax your knees and straighten them.
4. Draw your thighs up and slightly turn them in. Lift your kneecaps.
5. Lift the arches of the feet.
6. Straighten your tailbone, and relax your abdominal muscles.
7. Lift your chest so that it is forward. Expand your shoulders outward, and relax them.
8. Feel your breathing as you inhale and exhale.

9. Inhale and lift your toes, transferring the weight to your heels.
10. Stretch your chest and arms upwards.
11. Stretch your neck.
12. Feel the stretch in your body.
13. Remain in the pose for one minute.

Benefits
- Improves posture
- Promotes blood circulation
- Firms the shoulders and thighs
- Strengthens the legs
- Develops stillness
- Improves focus
- Calms the mind

Caution
Avoid practicing the pose if you have low blood pressure. Do not practice the pose while experiencing headache or dizziness.

Half Wheel Pose

Half wheel pose is an ideal pose for beginners to learn balance and prepare the body for advanced backbends.

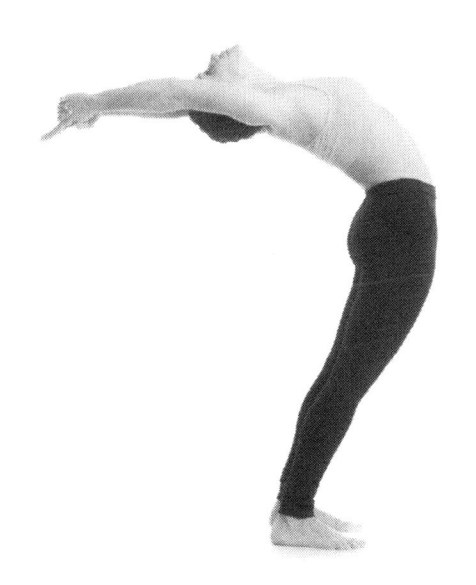

Instructions
1. Stand, placing your feet together. Let your hands rest by your sides.
2. Keep your spine erect.
3. Inhale as you lift your arms over your head, and bend your body backwards. Your arms should go proportionately back with your torso.
4. Keep the knees straight and arch your back so the pelvis comes forward.
5. You can bring the palms together or you can keep them parallel to each other.
6. Remain in the pose for 30 seconds.
7. Exhale and stand straight as you come out of the pose.

Benefits
- Stretches the spine and improves spine flexibility
- Tones and strengthens the back
- Relieves back pain
- Relieves tension in the neck
- Expands the shoulders and chest
- Improves lung function
- Maintains healthy blood pressure
- Reduces the symptoms of spondylitis
- Stimulates the function of the abdominal organs
- Reduces excess fat in the hips
- Relieves menstrual disorders

Note
Beginners can keep their hands on their hips until they acquire balance.

Caution
Avoid practicing this pose if you have severe spinal problems.

Standing Spinal Twist Pose

Standing Spinal twist pose involves gentle rotation of the waist. It is highly recommended for beginners who have just begun developing their flexibility.

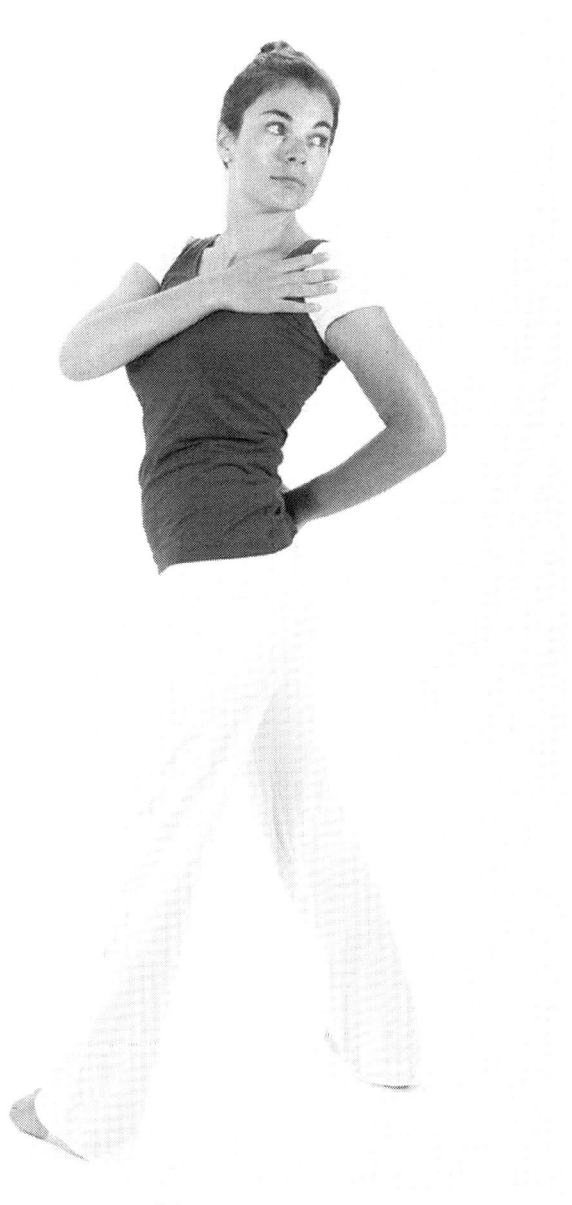

Instructions
1. Stand straight with your feet about shoulder width apart.
2. Inhale, twist, and cross your right arm over the body to place the palm on the left shoulder.
3. Slide the left arm behind you and bring it over to the right side of your back.
4. Exhale as you twist your torso to your left without bending your knees. Keep your spine straight.
5. Turn your head to look over your left shoulder.
6. Remain in the pose for 30 seconds.
7. Come out of the pose by turning your torso to the front with an inhale.
8. Repeat the same process on the other side.

Benefits
- Stretches the shoulders, spine, and back
- Improves flexibility of the upper torso.
- Promotes blood supply to the midsection
- Tones the waist

Lateral Half Moon Pose

Lateral half moon pose makes your hips flexible. The pose involves bending to the sides.

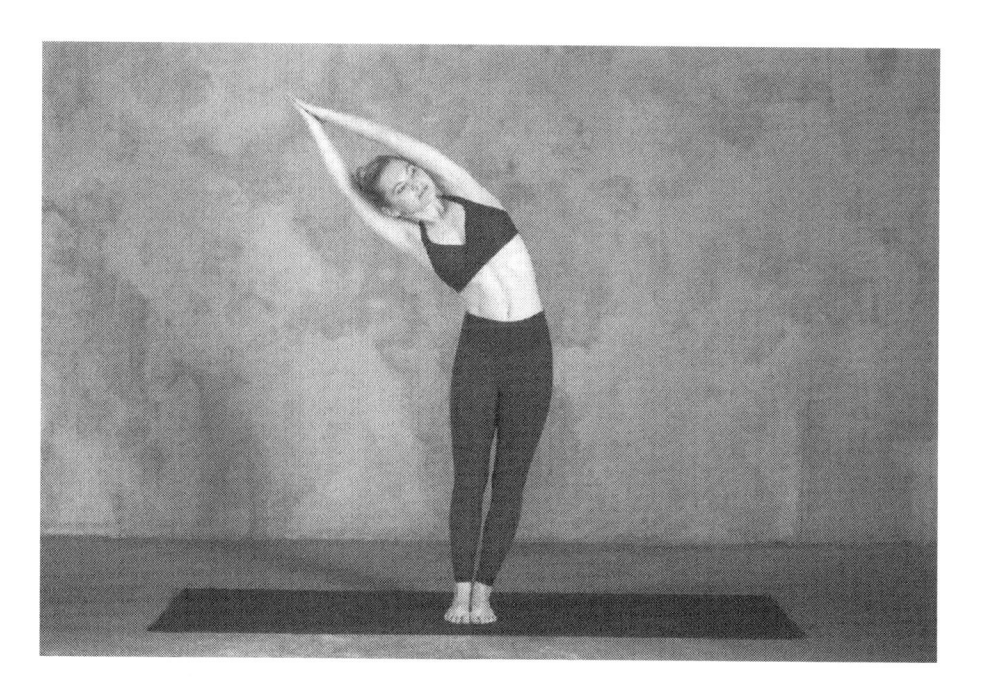

Instructions
1. Stand straight with your feet together and your hands by your sides.
2. Inhale as you slowly raise your right hand over your head without bending the elbow. The biceps of the right hand should be close to your ear.
3. Exhale as you bend sideways to your right. As you bend, your left hand will slide down, and your right arm will go sideways over the head pointing toward the left wall.
4. Remain in the pose for 30 seconds.
5. Repeat the same on the other side.

Benefits
- Improves hip flexibility
- Stretches the arms and shoulders
- Improves lung function
- Reduces fat in the tummy and waist
- Relieves constipation

Note

As you bend to one side, your hips should straight. Do not lean forward or backward.

Caution

Avoid practicing this pose if you have a hip injury.

Double Angle Pose

Double angle pose is a gentle forward bend, ideal for beginners.

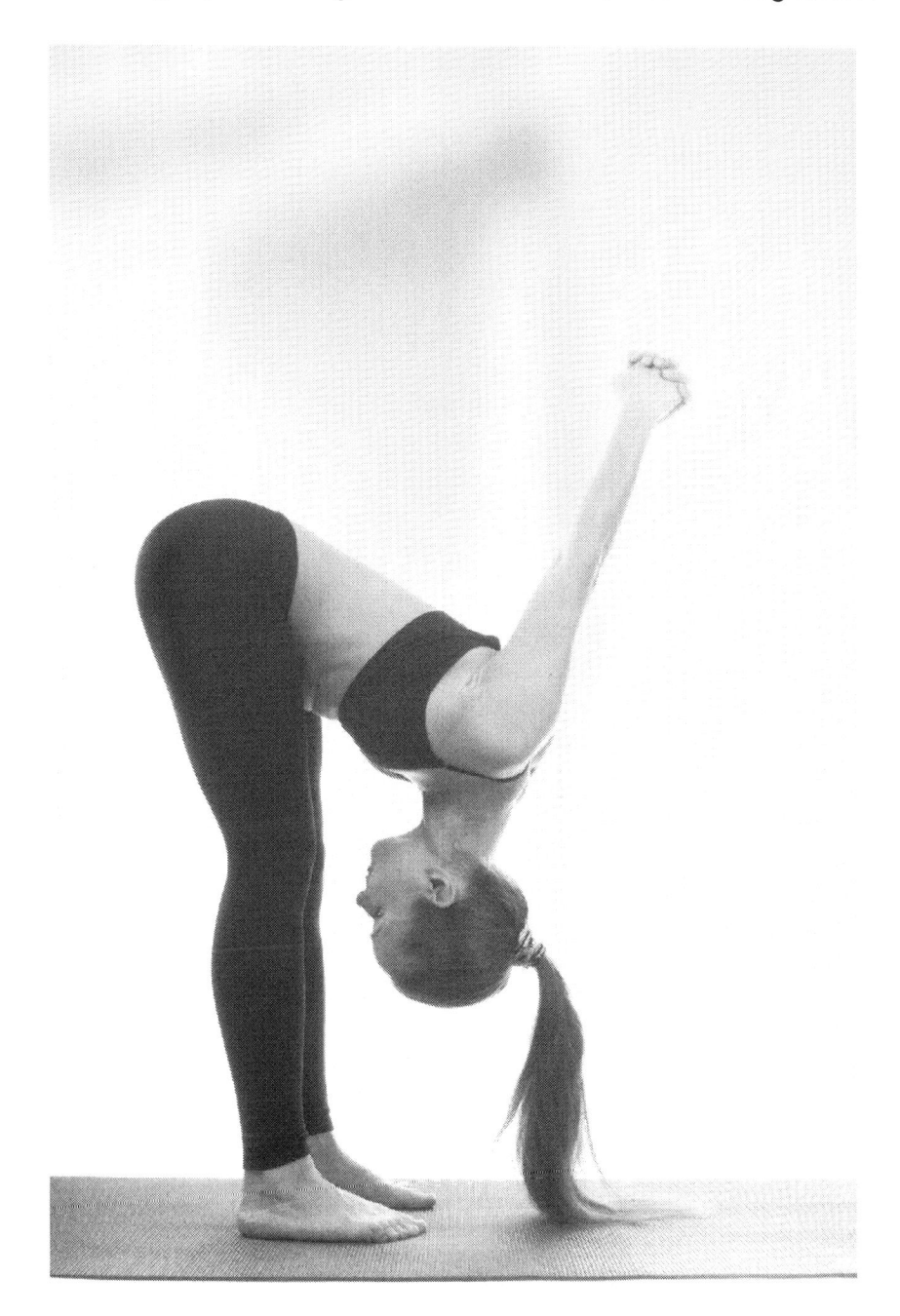

Instruction
1. Stand straight. Keep your feet about shoulder width apart.
2. Bring your hands behind you, and interlock the fingers.
3. Exhale as you bend forward. Keep your torso parallel to the ground.
4. Raise your arms so they are perpendicular to your torso.
5. Remain in the pose for 30 seconds.
6. Inhale as you straighten your torso and lower your arms.

Benefits
- Strengthens the back and hips
- Stretches the chest, shoulders, and arms
- Stretches the back of the thighs

Gate Pose

Gate pose works on the sides of the body, and complements the results produced by other side bending poses.

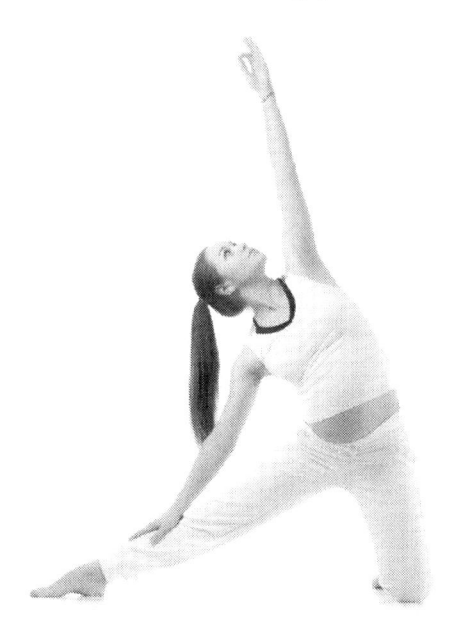

Instructions

1. Kneel down on the floor. Your knees should be aligned with your hips.
2. Extend your right leg towards your right side. Place the right foot on the ground, keeping the leg straight without shifting the position of the body.
3. Place your right palm on the outer side of the right thigh.
4. With inhalation, stretch your left arm up, keeping the fingers pointing the ceiling. Keep the palm turned to the right and the forearm close to left ear.
5. Exhaling, bend to your right. Keep the shoulders straight.
6. As you bend, slide your right hand down the right leg.
7. Turn your head upwards in the left direction gazing at the space past your left elbow.
8. Remain in the pose for 30 seconds.
9. Repeat the same steps with the other leg and hand.

Benefits
- Stretches the spine and tones the back muscles
- Stretches the sides of the body and neck
- Opens the shoulders
- Stimulates the lungs and improves lung performance
- Boosts the function of the abdominal organs
- Stretches the legs

Note
If placing the sole of the extended foot on the ground is difficult, you can place your leg on a yoga block or against a wall. Those with a knee injury can perform this pose while seated on a chair.

Caution
Those with severe injuries to the hips should refrain from practicing this pose.

Goddess Pose

Also called fierce angle pose, goddess pose is a mild, core-stretching pose for beginners.

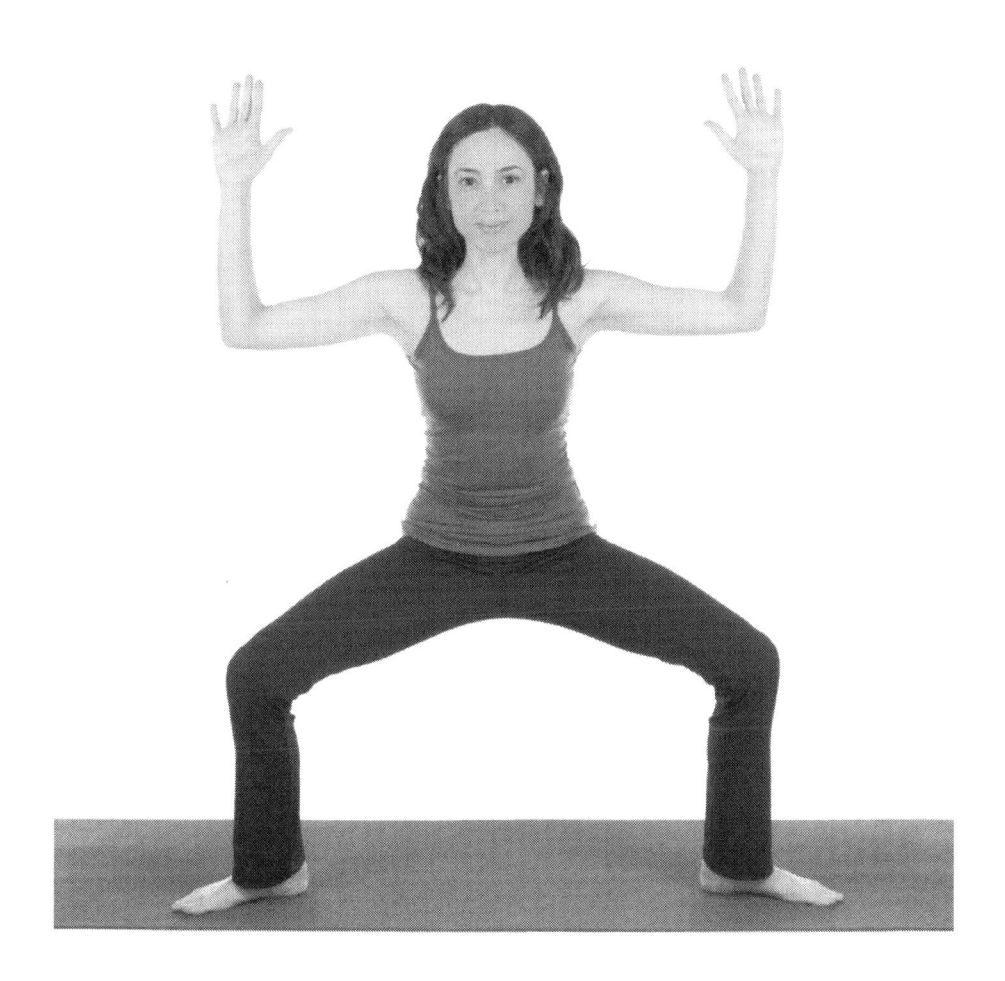

Instructions
1. Stand straight with your legs together and your hands by your sides.
2. Step your feet wide. Maintain a distance of about three feet between your feet.
3. Turn your feet slightly outwards, so your toes point towards the corners of the yoga mat.
4. Exhale as you lower your body to squat with your knees in line with your toes. Your thighs should be parallel to the ground.
5. Stretch your arms out sideways at shoulder level. Your thumbs should be upwards, and your palms should face forward.
6. Bend your elbows, and raise your forearms up so the fingertips are pointing at the ceiling. Keep the forearms elbow distance apart.
7. Gaze straight ahead.
8. Remain in the pose for 30 seconds.
9. Come out of the pose by bringing your feet together and lowering your hands to your sides.

Benefits
- Stretches the spine and tones the back
- Strengthens the hips and legs
- Expands the chest and improves respiratory function
- Strengthens the heart
- Supports natural childbirth
- Energizes the whole body

Note
Beginners can practice this pose against a wall. Instead of raising the forearms, you can place your palms on a support.

Caution
Avoid practicing the pose if you have chronic injury in shoulders, back, hips, or legs.

Corpse Pose

Corpse pose is the best relaxation pose in yoga. The pose is often performed after challenging yoga poses and towards the end of the yoga session. It may seem like the simplest pose to perform, but it can be challenging to keep the mind tuned towards the pose. Any yoga session is incomplete without performing the corpse pose.

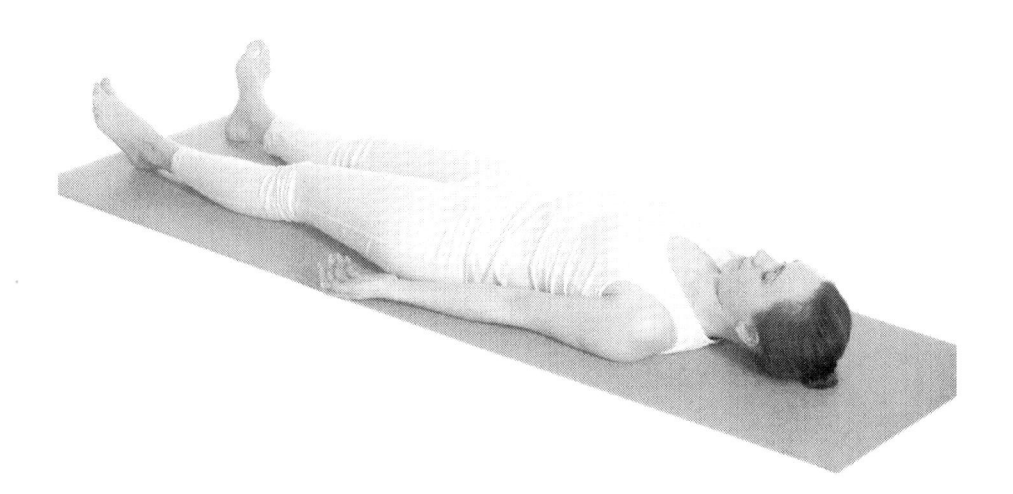

Instructions
1. Lie on your back, keeping your legs apart. Your hands should be slightly away from your sides. Keep your eyes closed.
2. Inhale and exhale slowly and deeply.
3. Starting from your toes, focus on every part of your body, working your way up and relaxing every part as you go.
4. If your mind wanders away, gently draw it to your body. Observe every part of the body mentally. If you feel tightness or tension anywhere, relax that area.

5. Watch your breath. Observe the changes in your body with every inhale and exhale.
6. Remain in the pose for about 10 minutes, or increase the duration based on your physical and psychological needs.
7. Come out of the pose by rolling over to your right. Place your left arm on the floor in front of your chest and sit in easy pose, in which you cross your legs and keep your hands on your knees.
8. With the eyes closed, take deep breaths. As you begin to be more aware of your surroundings, open your eyes.

Benefits

- Rejuvenates and relaxes the body and mind
- Brings your mind to a meditative state
- Normalizes blood pressure
- Promotes quality sleep
- Relieves headache
- Relieves nervous tension
- Relieves anxiety
- Cures fatigue
- Promotes self-confidence
- Boosts concentration
- Improves memory
- Calms your mind

Note

If lying on the floor for considerable time hurts your neck, keep your head elevated slightly by placing a folded blanket underneath.

Eight-Limbed Pose

Eight-Limbed pose is a basic pose which is done lying down. It is part of the Sun Salutation sequence.

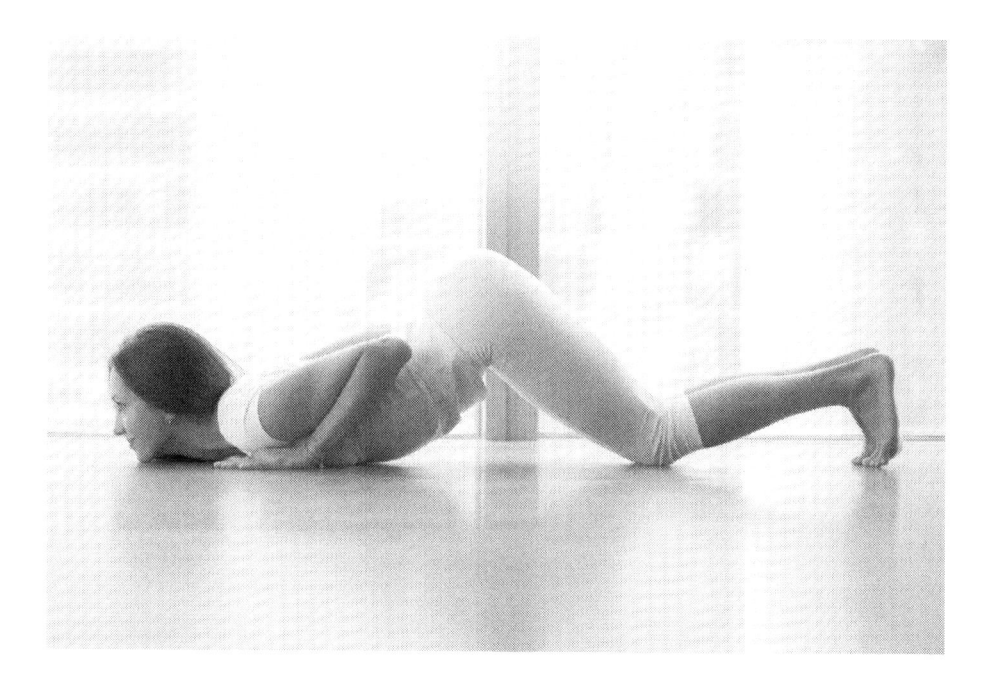

Instructions
1. Lie face down on the floor. Keep your arms by your sides.
2. Bend your hands and place your elbows on the floor close to your chest. Keeping your knees on the floor, lift your tailbone towards the ceiling.
3. Remain in the pose for 30 seconds.

Benefits
- Stretches the neck and shoulders
- Strengthens the arms
- Stretches the spine and tones the back
- Tones the hips

Caution
Those with any injury to the neck, shoulders, elbows, wrists, or back should refrain from practicing the pose.

Basic Poses for Strengthening the Arms

When we think of strengthening the arms, what comes to mind are exercises that may include lifting weights. Many people are aware that yoga makes you flexible, but don't realize it makes you stronger, too. Instead of weights, in yoga we build strength by supporting the body itself.

Here are the top yoga poses for strengthening your arms.

Reverse Table Top Pose

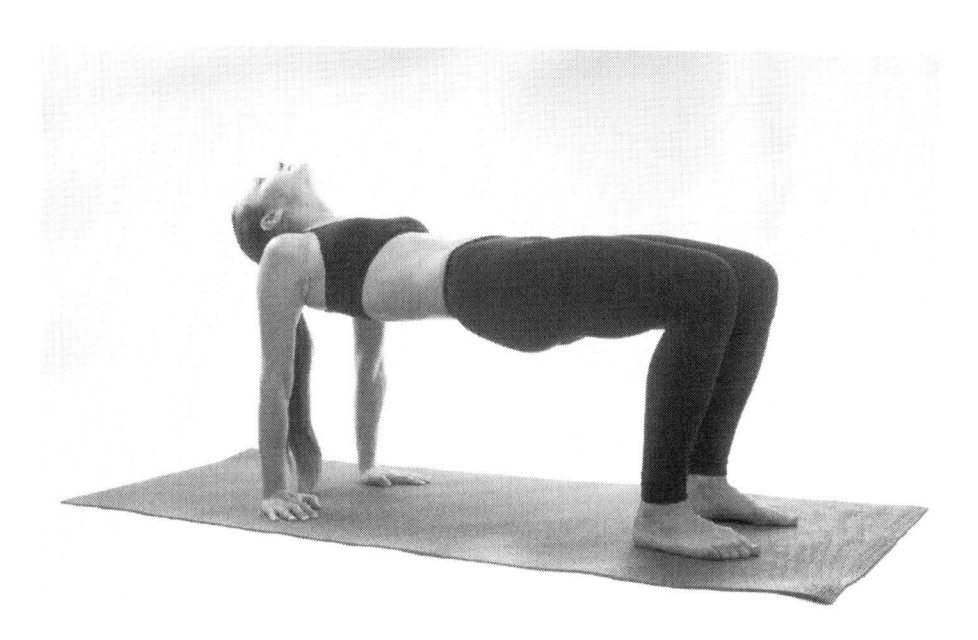

Instructions
1. Sit down with your legs stretched forward, and your arms by your sides.
2. Bend your legs and place your feet on the ground.
3. Maintain hip-width distance between your feet.

4. Place your palms behind your buttocks, but not too close. The hands should be shoulder-width apart.
5. With the hands and legs pressed firmly on the ground, lift your hips up until you are in one straight line from chest to knees.
6. Your palms should be below your shoulders and your feet below your knees.
7. Gently let your head drop down so you can see the wall behind you.
8. Relax your shoulders, and then the entire body.
9. Remain in the pose for 30 seconds.

Benefits
- Opens the chest
- Stretches the shoulders, abdomen, and spine
- Tones and strengthens the arms
- Boosts respiratory function
- Strengthens the core muscles and legs
- Promotes balance
- Relieves fatigue

Note
You can keep your head straight if dropping it back causes discomfort.

Caution
The pose is not recommended for those with carpal tunnel syndrome, or other injury in the wrists or shoulders. Those with neck pain should also avoid practicing the pose.

Cobra Pose

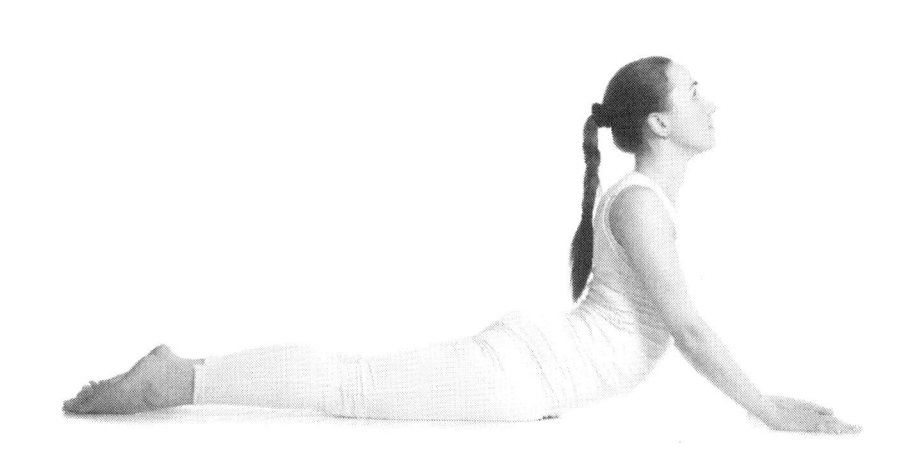

Instructions

1. Lie down on your stomach with your legs extended. Keep your hands by your sides.
2. Keep the tops of your feet on the mat.
3. Place your palms by the sides of your chest, close to your shoulders on the mat. Your elbows should be pointing upwards, and your shoulders should be drawn back.
4. Inhale as you lift your chest and head off the floor.
5. If you are comfortable, you can lift your torso further up until your arms straighten.
6. Lift your chin up to fix your gaze above you. If that is too uncomfortable, you can look straight ahead instead.
7. Remain in the pose for 30 seconds.

Benefits

- Stimulates your spine and increases spine flexibility
- Tones the upper back muscles
- Strengthens the shoulders and arms

- Boosts lung function and relieves respiratory conditions, including asthma
- Tones the abdomen and supports the healthy function of the abdominal organs
- Improves digestion
- Relieves fatigue
- Stimulates Kundalini (spiritual energy which is said to originate at the base of the spine)

Note

If you initially find the pose tough to perform, you can perform the pose standing against a wall, pressing away from it with your palms.

Caution

Those with health conditions such as carpal tunnel syndrome, peptic ulcer, and wrist injury should not practice this pose. It is also not recommended if you have recently undergone abdominal surgery.

Plank Pose

Also called Utthita Caturanga Dandasana, plank pose is an arm balancing pose, and one of the best poses for beginners to promote arm strength.

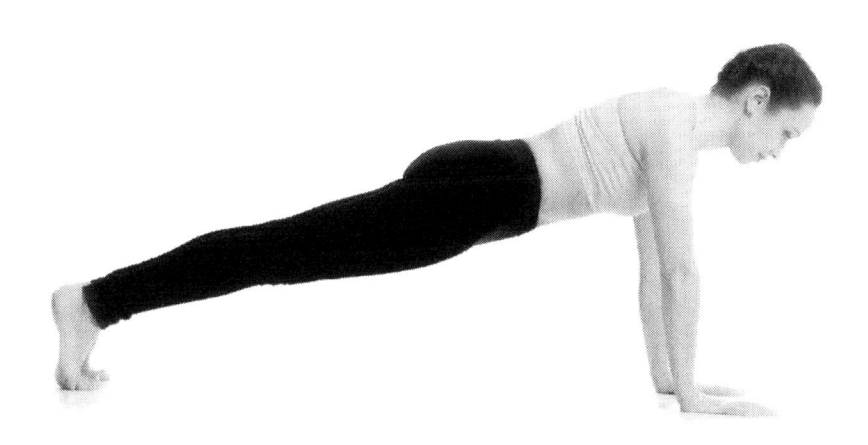

Instructions
1. Place your palms and knees on the mat. Your palms should be aligned with your shoulders.
2. Lift your knees off the ground and extend your legs backwards, stretching fully so your body is in a straight line. Keep the toes tucked in.
3. Look down at the space between your hands.
4. Hold the pose for one minute. When that becomes easy, you can increase the duration up to five minutes.

Benefits
- Strengthens the shoulders, arms, and wrists
- Strengthens the spine, core muscles, and back muscles
- Stimulates the nervous system
- Builds stamina
- Promotes endurance

Note

If performing the pose is difficult due to a lack of strength in your arms and abdomen, you can rest your knees on the mat. Once your strength improves, you can practice the pose to perfection.

Caution

Avoid performing the pose if you have osteoporosis. Those with carpal tunnel syndrome can perform the pose with knees or forearms down (see dolphin plank pose).

Intermediate Poses for Strengthening Arms

Dolphin Plank Pose

Dolphin plank pose is a variation of plank pose.

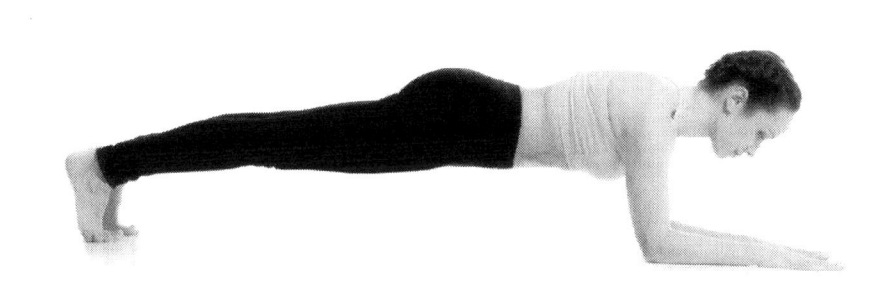

Instructions
1. Begin in downward dog pose, in which you are on your palms and feet resembling an inverted 'V'.
2. Draw your body forward so your shoulders are in line with your wrists, and your heels above your toes.
3. Bend your arms to place your forearms on the floor. Your elbows should be directly under your shoulders.
4. Keep your knees straight.
5. Gaze at the floor between your forearms.
6. Breathe normally.
7. Remain in the pose for one minute.

Benefits
- Strengthens the arms
- Stretches and strengthens the legs
- Stimulates the function of the abdominal organs
- Cures some types of back pain
- Relieves pain during the menstrual cycle
- Relieves fatigue

Note
Beginners can place their knees on the floor while performing the asana. With practice, the pose can be perfected.

Caution
Those with an injury to the neck, spine, and back should perform the pose with support and under expert supervision.

Upward Facing Dog Pose

Upward facing dog is an excellent intermediate pose for strengthening the arms.

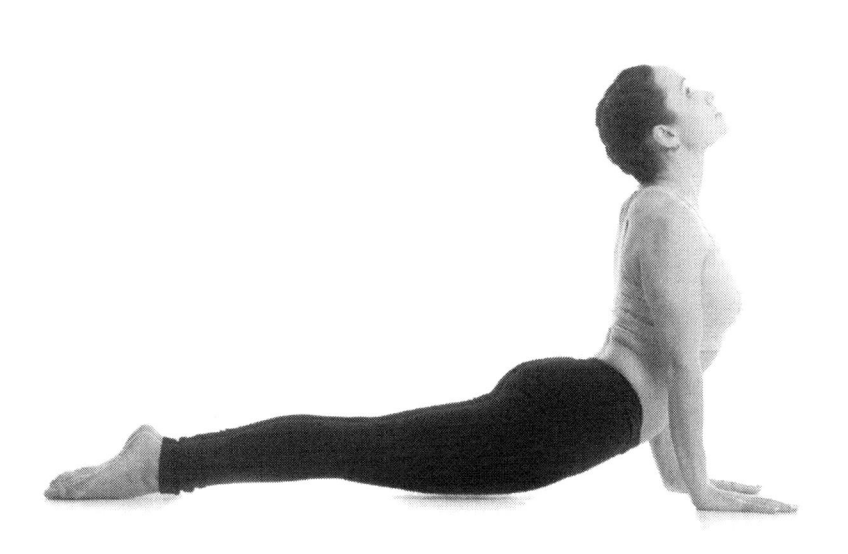

Instructions
1. Lie down on your front on the floor. Stretch your legs long, with few inches of space between your feet, and keep your hands by your sides. Keep the toes pointed backwards so the tops of your feet are on the floor.
2. Place your palms by the sides of your body, keeping the elbows close to ribcage. Let the fingers be pointed forward.
3. With inhalation, keep your palms firmly on the floor, and arms stretched straight out to the front. Lift your torso and your legs off the floor so only the tops of your feet and your palms are on the floor. Look upwards.
4. Remain in the pose for 30 to 60 seconds.
5. Come out of the pose by placing your knees on the floor and drawing your torso back to sit on your heels, or to perform child's pose (sitting on your knees, palms on your thighs).

Benefits
- Opens the chest and improves respiratory function
- Strengthens the shoulders, arms, wrists, and legs
- Stretches the spine and tones the back
- Corrects posture
- Relieves back pain
- Relieves sciatic pain
- Stretches and energizes the whole body
- Strengthens the nervous system
- Stimulates the function of abdominal organs
- Improves digestion
- Relieves fatigue
- Cures mild depression

Note
If holding the thighs away from the floor is difficult, place a folded blanket below your hips.

Caution
Upward facing dog pose is not recommended for those with carpal tunnel syndrome, or injury in the shoulders, wrists, back, or hip.

Elevated Lotus Pose

Elevated lotus pose is a more advanced version of lotus pose. The pose is highly effective in strengthening arms.

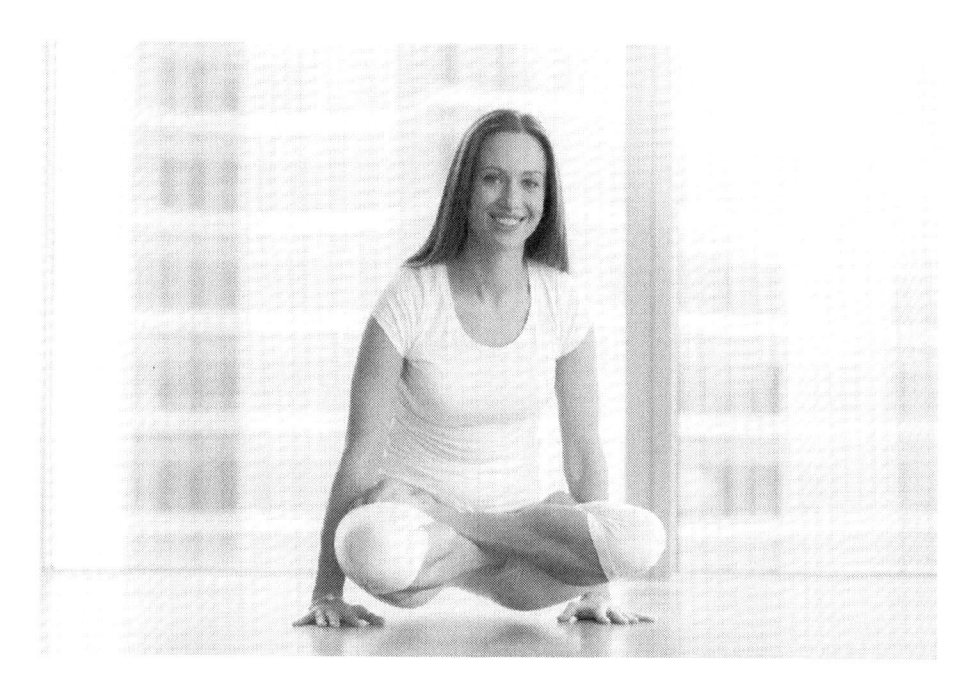

Instructions
1. Sit in lotus pose.
2. Keep your hands on the floor by your hips.
3. Exhale, press the palms firmly on the floor, and lift your body off the floor. Your arms should be vertical, and not slanted outwards.
4. Remain in the pose for 30 seconds.
5. Inhale as you come out of the pose by sitting on the floor and releasing your legs and hands.

Benefits
- Strengthens the arms and wrists.
- Strengthens the shoulders
- Improves respiratory function

- Opens the hips
- Tones the back
- Strengthens the abdominal muscles
- Stimulates the function of the abdominal organs
- Reduces tummy fat
- Promotes a sense of balance
- Calms your mind

Note
If performing elevated lotus pose while keeping your legs crossed is difficult, perform the pose in half lotus position. You will lift your buttocks off the floor with the lower legs on the floor.

Caution
Do not perform the pose if you have severe knee or ankle problems. It is also not recommended for those with chronic hip problems.

Basic Poses for Stretching and Strengthening the Legs

For people who don't go to a gym, one of the most ignored parts of the body is the leg. In spite of the weight legs carry, they are cared for only when they hurt. Keeping your legs healthy is important for your overall health. And for those who believe yoga is not for strengthening legs, here are some reasons to reconsider.

- Yoga stretches and strengthens muscles in every part of the body, including the legs.
- Standing yoga poses strengthen leg muscles, increase balance, and promote stability.
- Yoga improves flexibility in the legs, which contributes not only to legs being healthy, but also strong.
- Yoga strengthens and tightens muscles around the knees, to better support them.
- Certain poses lengthen the legs, release tension, and promote good health.

Hence, yoga builds strength; not only core strength but also overall strength including leg strength. Here are the top yoga poses for stretching and strengthening your legs.

Chair Pose

Chair pose strengthens your thigh muscles, calf muscles, and ankles. Regular practice of the pose builds stamina and strength.

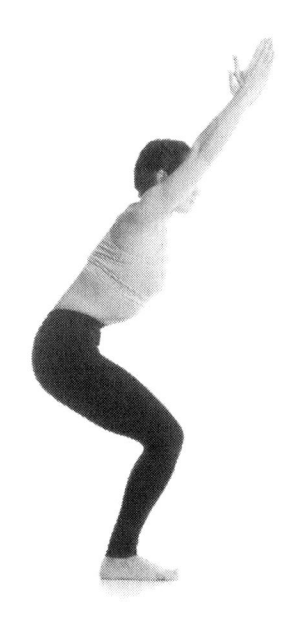

Instructions
1. Stand straight with your feet together. Beginners can place the feet hip-width apart. Keep your arms by your sides.
2. Inhale as you lift your hands over your head. Keep your hands perpendicular to the floor without bending the elbows.
3. Alternately, you can stretch your hands straight out at shoulder level. With practice, you can lift your hands over your head and bring the palms together.
4. Exhale and lower your body by bending your knees.
5. Your thighs should be parallel to the ground, and your back arched slightly.

6. As you lower your body, feel as if you are sitting in an imaginary chair. This will help you to perfect the pose.
7. Expand your shoulders, and look straight ahead.
8. Remain in the pose for one minute.

Benefits

- Strengthens the legs and tones the leg muscles
- Strengthens the nervous system
- Promotes lung health
- Protects heart health; boosts blood circulation
- Stimulates the abdominal organs and improves their function
- Boosts endurance
- Stretches shoulders
- Tones the hips and back
- Reduces flat foot if practiced from an early age

Note

You can stand with your back close to a wall for support. As you lower your head, your tailbone should maintain only light contact with the wall to keep your pose stable. Once you are balanced, you can move away from the wall.

Caution

Those with a hip injury or low blood pressure should refrain from practicing this pose. Avoid practicing the pose while experiencing headache.

Standing Forward Bend

Standing forward bend is an excellent beginner yoga poses that promotes leg strength.

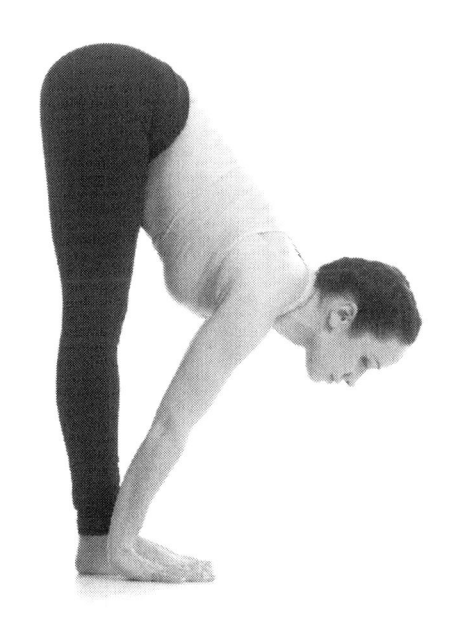

Instructions
1. Stand straight up with your feet together. Place your hands on your hips.
2. Exhale, and bend at your hips.
3. Stretch your spine to bend as low as possible without bending your knees.
4. Let your head hang down. You may also stretch your neck to lift your head, arching the back of your neck.
5. Place your palms on the floor by the sides of your feet, or behind your ankles.
6. Pull your thigh muscles up.
7. Remain in the pose for one minute.
8. While coming out of the pose, inhale, lift your upper body straight and bring your hands to your sides.

Benefits
- Stretches and strengthens the back of the legs from the thighs to calf muscles and ankles
- Strengthens the spine and promotes spine flexibility
- Relieves symptoms of asthma
- Improves osteoporosis symptoms
- Improves digestion
- Stimulates the function of the liver and kidneys
- Promotes fertility
- Reduces menopausal discomfort
- Relieves headache
- Reduces high blood pressure
- Cures insomnia
- Calms the mind
- Relieves depression

Note
Those with a back injury can perform the pose with bent knees.

Tree Pose

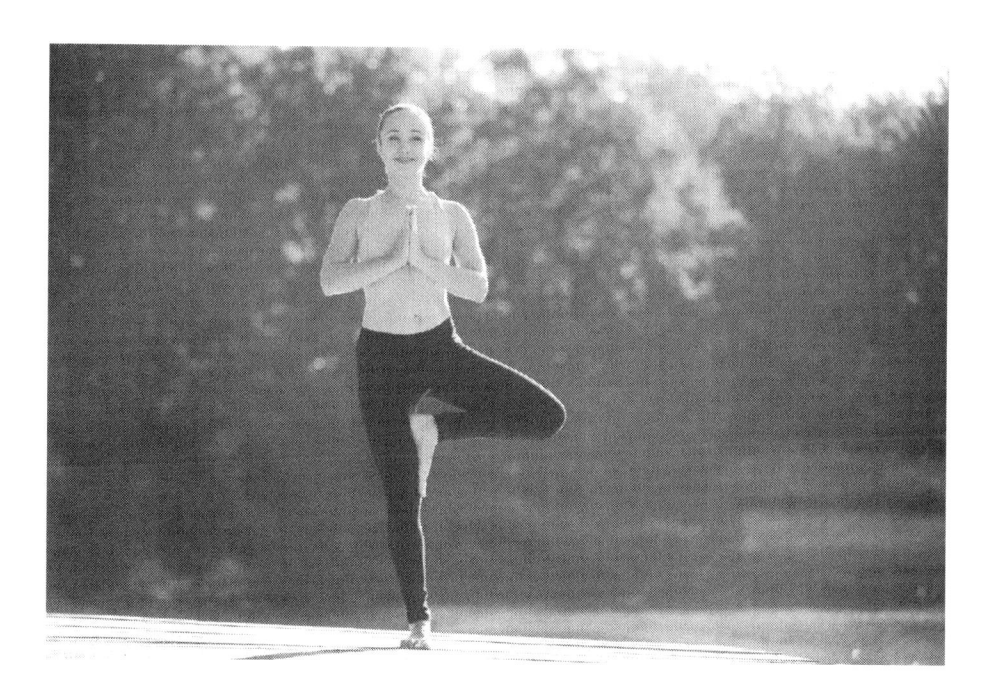

Instructions

1. Stand straight with the spine erect and your arms by your sides.
2. Hold your right ankle and place your right foot against the inner thigh of the left leg. The heel should press against the inner groin, and the toes should point downwards.
3. Press the right heel firmly against the left thigh while keeping the left leg straight.
4. Lift your hands sideways and over your head. Bring the palms together, keeping the elbows straight. You can also place your palms together in front of your chest.
5. Remain in the pose for one minute.
6. Repeat the same steps with the other leg.

Benefits
- Stretches the arms, legs, shoulders, and spine
- Strengthens the legs
- Relieves sciatica
- Strengthens the hip bones
- Helps with flat feet
- Postpones symptoms of aging
- Promotes balance
- Boosts concentration
- Promotes self-confidence

Note
If you find it difficult to hold the pose, use a wall for support until you gain stability.

Caution
Those with insomnia, low blood pressure, or severe knee or hip problems should avoid practicing the pose. It is also recommended to keep the hands down if you have high blood pressure.

Downward Facing Dog Pose

Downward facing dog pose is an excellent pose for beginners to tone leg muscles.

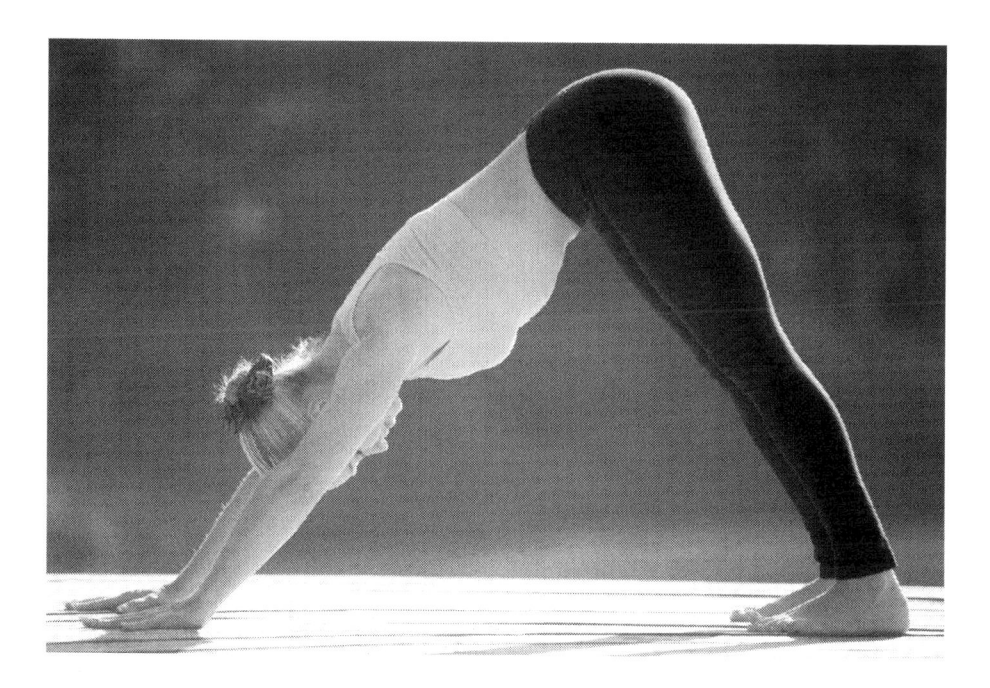

Instructions
1. Go on all fours with your palms and toes on the floor.
2. Align your wrists with your shoulders, and your knees with your hips.
3. Exhale as you lift your hips up towards the ceiling.
4. Stretch your hands fully.
5. Stretch your legs and place your heels on the floor (or as close as you can).
6. Tuck in your head and fix your gaze on your navel. Now you will resemble an inverted 'V' shape.
7. Remain in the pose for one minute.

Benefits
- Energizes the whole body
- Stretches the shoulders, spine and legs
- Relieves symptoms of asthma
- Tones the back and relieves back pain
- Relieves headache
- Reduces menopausal symptoms
- Prevents osteoporosis
- Postpones symptoms of aging
- Effective for flat feet
- Helps cure insomnia
- Calms the brain
- Relieves stress

Note
If you find placing your feet on the floor difficult, you can keep your toes down. With practice you will be able to keep your feet flat.

Caution
Avoid practicing the pose if you have high blood pressure. Those with chronic back conditions and carpal tunnel syndrome should avoid downward dog. Do not perform the pose if your eyes or ears are infected.

High Lunge Pose

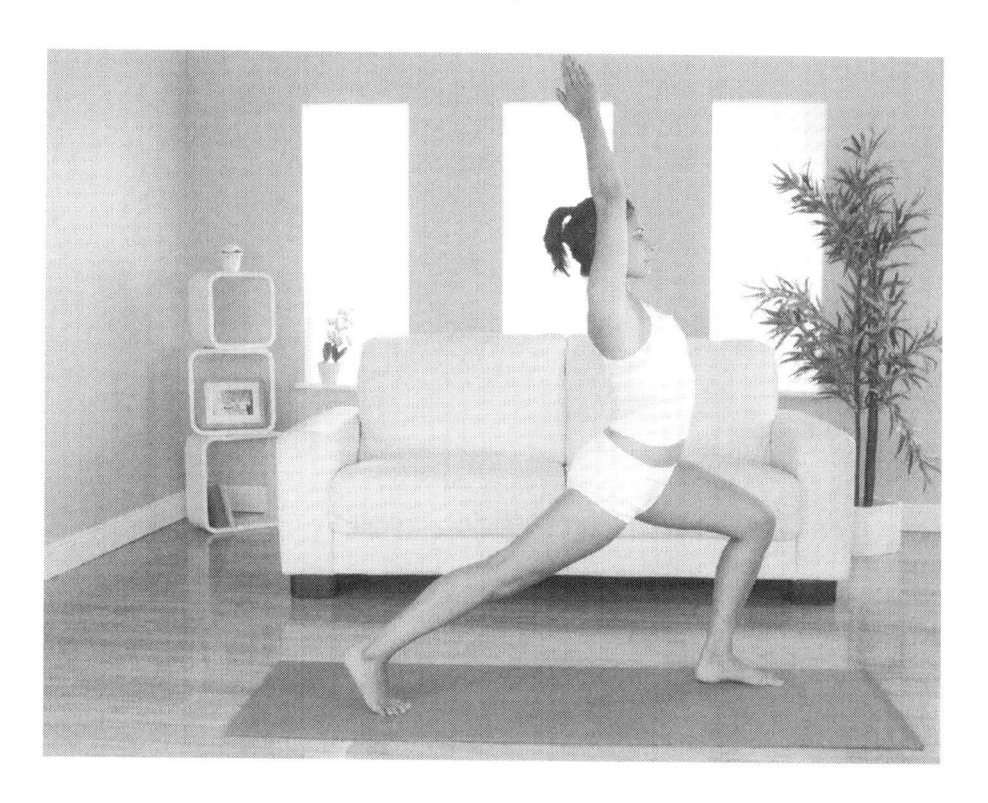

Instructions
1. Go into downward dog pose.
2. Bring your right knee towards your face, placing your right foot between your palms.
3. Lift your left heel off the floor. Lift your face and fix your gaze straight ahead.
4. Balance your weight on your knees, lift your torso up, and stretch your hands up.
5. Your right calf should be perpendicular to the floor.
6. Remain in the pose for one minute.

Benefits
- Relieves constipation
- Cures indigestion
- Strengthens the legs and arms

- Lengthens the spine
- Opens the chest and hips
- Strengthens the lower body
- Relieves sciatic pain

Caution

Those with any knee or back injury should refrain from practicing this pose.

Warrior Pose I

The difference between high lunge pose and warrior pose I is that in high lunge you lift the heel of the back leg, whereas in Warrior I, you place the back heel on the floor.

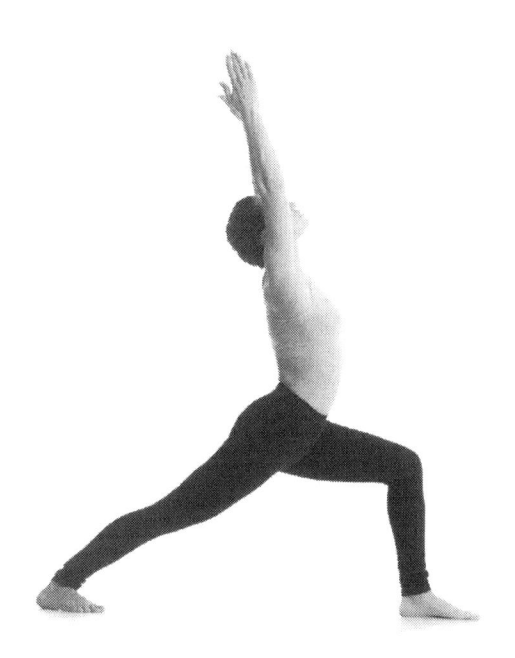

Instructions
1. Stand straight with your hands by your sides.
2. Exhale, lift your left leg, and place the left foot about four feet behind you.
3. Bend your right leg until the thigh is parallel to the floor.
4. Turn your left foot 90 degrees to your left, so your feet are perpendicular to each other.
5. Raise your arms up close to your ears, with the palms facing each other. Look straight ahead.
6. If you would like to deepen your pose, bring your palms together. Arch your back a little and lift your head to look above you.
7. Remain in the pose for 30 seconds.
8. Repeat with the right leg at the back.

Benefits
- Energizes the whole body
- Boosts respiratory function
- Strengthens the leg muscles and feet
- Strengthens the shoulders and arms
- Promotes core strength
- Tones the spine and back muscles
- Improves coordination and balance
- Promotes focus
- Develops confidence

Note
If lifting the hands is difficult initially, you may place your hands on your hips.

Caution
Avoid performing the pose if you have a back, hip, or knee injury. Those with a shoulder injury can keep their hands down or on hips.

Warrior Pose II

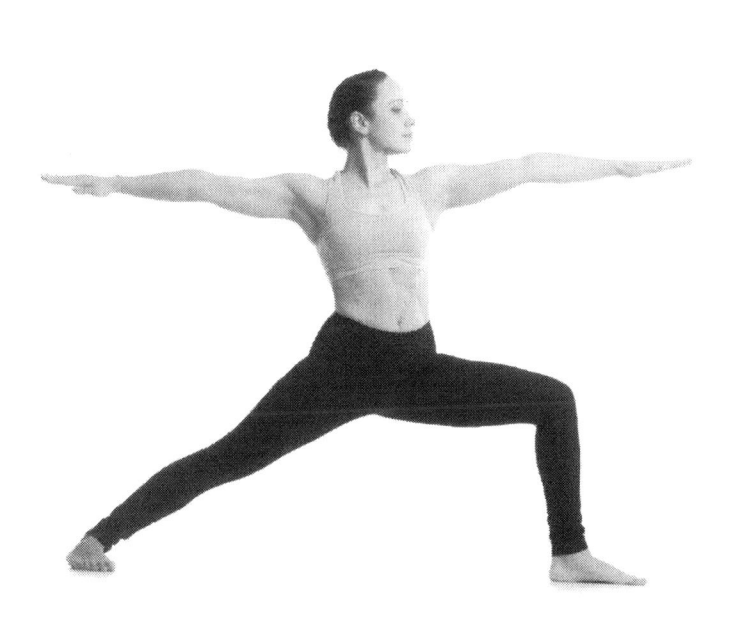

Instructions
1. Stand straight. Keep your feet slightly apart.
2. Bring your right leg forward and place it on the floor about five feet apart from left leg, or as far as you can. The toes of your right foot should be pointed forward.
3. Turn your left foot outward, so the heels are aligned under you, front to back.
4. Lift your hands to shoulder level. Extend your right hand to the front over your thigh, and your left hand behind. Your wrists should be in line with your ankles.
5. Bend your right knee until your right thigh becomes parallel to the floor.
6. Look at the fingers of your right hand, stretched forward.
7. Remain in the pose for one minute.
8. Repeat the same procedure on the other side.

Benefits
- Stretches and strengthens the legs
- Stretches the arms and shoulders
- Opens the chest and hips
- Boosts lung function
- Tones the back and relieves back pain
- Stimulates the function of the abdominal organs
- Energizes the body
- Promotes blood circulation
- Improves fertility
- Improves focus
- Promotes balance

Note
You can place your hands on your hips if you have difficulty stretching your arms out.

Caution
Those with high blood pressure, or an injury to the shoulder, hips, or knees should refrain from practicing this pose. Do not perform the pose when you are experiencing diarrhea.

Garland Pose

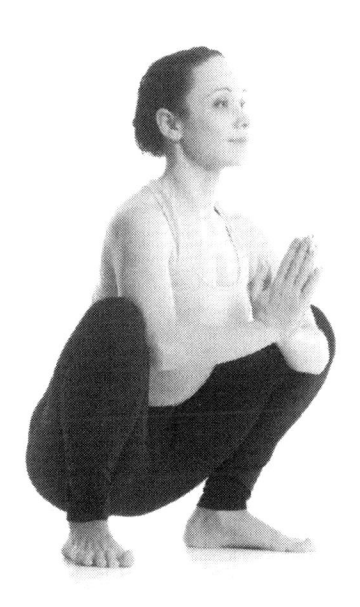

Instructions
1. Go into a squat position, keeping your feet flat on the floor.
2. Move your thighs apart, and lean forward to fit your torso in the space between them.
3. Place your elbows against the inner knees, bringing your palms together and gently pushing the knees away.
4. Remain in the pose for one minute.

Benefits
- Strengthens the spine
- Strengthens the thighs, ankles, and calves
- Increases knee and ankle flexibility
- Opens your hips
- Tones the abdominal muscles and improves digestion
- Reduces tummy fat
- Relieves constipation
- Boosts metabolism

Note
If you are unable to squat low, you may sit on a chair.

Caution
Those with any knee injury or lower back pain should avoid doing this pose.

Intermediate Poses for Strengthening Legs

Intense Side Stretch

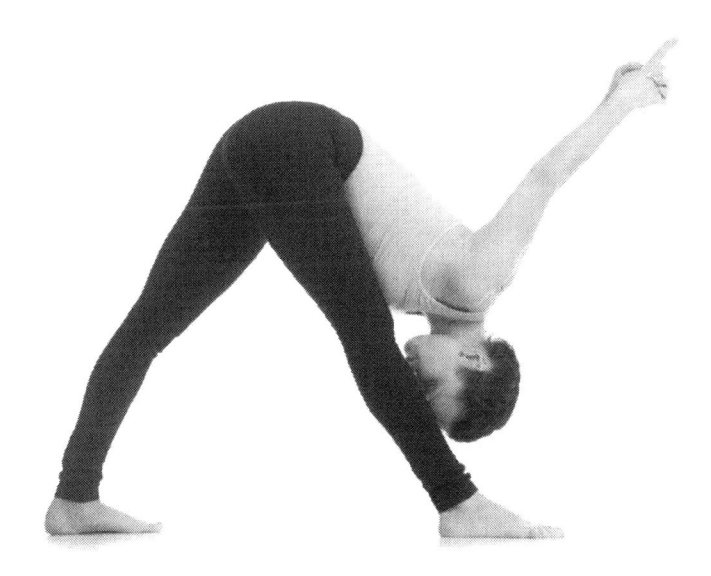

Instructions
1. Stand straight with your arms by your sides, feet together.
2. Exhale, and place your feet apart from each other, maintaining a distance of about 4 feet.
3. Turn your right foot to the right, and your left foot slightly toward the right. The heels should be aligned under you.
4. Place your hands on your hips.
5. Exhale as your turn your torso to the right.
6. Inhale. Slide your hands behind your back and place the palms against each other, as though in prayer. You may also interlock your fingers and stretch your hands behind your back.

7. Exhale, and bend forward at the hips so your torso is over the right thigh, and your face over your knee or below. The arms extend upwards.
8. Remain in the pose for 30 seconds.
9. Repeat the same steps on the other side.

Benefits
- Stretches and strengthens the legs
- Stretches the spine
- Tones the back muscles
- Stretches the shoulders and hips
- Opens the hips
- Stimulates the abdominal organs
- Improves digestion
- Improves flat feet
- Promotes balance
- Calms the brain

Note
If you are unable to do reverse prayer with hands behind your back, place the tips of your fingers on the ground. You may also bring your hands behind you, and hold the opposite elbows.

Caution
Those with high blood pressure or back conditions should perform the pose under professional guidance.

Revolved Side Angle Pose

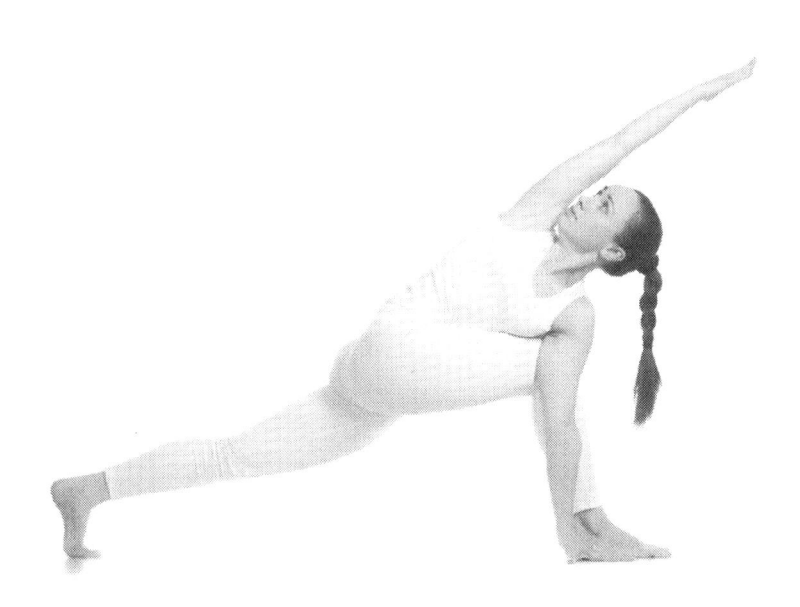

Instructions
1. Stand straight, keeping your feet four to five feet apart. Keep your arms by your sides.
2. Turn your right foot towards the right at a 90 degree angle. Turn your left foot towards the right as well, at an angle of 45 degrees.
3. Turn your torso in the direction of your right leg.
4. Bend your right knee. Your knee should be in line with your ankle, and perpendicular to the floor.
5. Inhale as you lift your arms sideways and overhead.
6. Place your palms together and lower them to your chest.
7. Twist your torso to your right. Lean forward towards the bent right knee, until your left elbow is on the outer side of your right thigh.
8. Your chest should be facing to your right.

9. Stretch your arms and place your left hand on the floor on the outer side of your right foot. Stretch your right arm over your head so your right bicep is close to your right ear. Your fingers should be pointing the direction your toes of the right leg are pointing.
10. Lengthen your spine.
11. Fix your gaze at the ceiling.
12. Remain in the pose for one minute.

Benefits

- Strengthens the spine, back, shoulders, and arms
- Stretches and strengthens the legs and ankles
- Opens the chest, improves lung capacity
- Stimulates the abdominal organs
- Builds stamina
- Aids in detoxification
- Energizes the whole body
- Strengthens the waist
- Improves flexibility
- Relieves sciatica
- Improves co-ordination of your body
- Boosts concentration levels
- Promotes balance

Note
If lifting the head towards the ceiling causes discomfort, you may look straight ahead instead.

Caution
Those with high or low blood pressure, severe back or neck injury, or insomnia should refrain from practicing this pose. Avoid practicing the pose if you have a headache.

Warrior Pose III

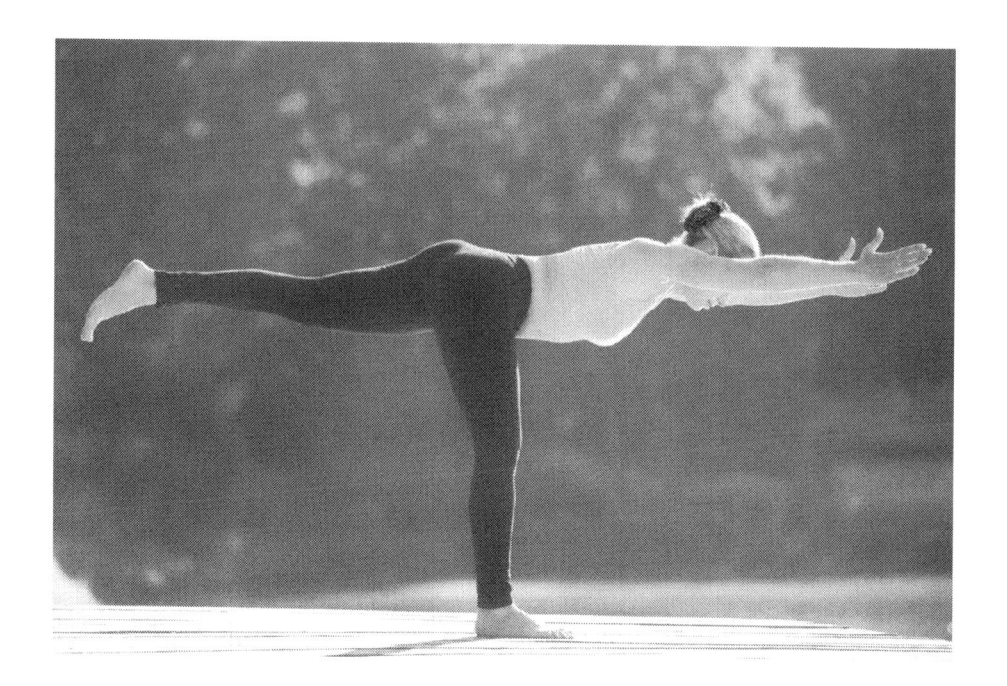

Instructions
1. Stand straight with your arms by your sides.
2. Place your right foot forward about twelve inches.
3. Pressing the right leg firmly to the floor, inhale, raise your arms over your head, and interlock your fingers.
4. Exhale, and lift your left leg. Bending at the hips, lower your torso and hands towards the ground. Your left leg, back, crown, and the extended arms should be in a straight line.
5. Keep your gaze fixed downward.
6. Remain in the pose for 30 seconds.
7. To come out of the pose, inhale as you lower your left leg to the ground. Straighten up your body and bring the hands down to the sides.

Benefits
- Improves balance
- Stretches and strengthens the legs and ankles
- Energizes the whole body
- Strengthens the spine, neck, shoulders, and back
- Builds stamina
- Tones abdominal organs and improves digestion
- Corrects posture

Note
If balancing is difficult, use a wall to lightly support your stretched fingers.

Caution
Those with an injury to the shoulders, spine, back, hips, or legs should refrain from practicing this pose.

Basic Poses for Strengthening the Shoulders

Studies have proven that shoulder pain is prevalent around the globe. Being a high-mobility joint, they are prone to injuries. Shoulder pain is also caused by various factors including poor posture, excess strain, shoulder joint instability, frozen shoulder, and osteoporosis. Strengthening your shoulders can help prevent these factors and keep your shoulders mobile. Many yoga poses promote shoulder strength and prevent health conditions associated with them.

Big Toe Pose

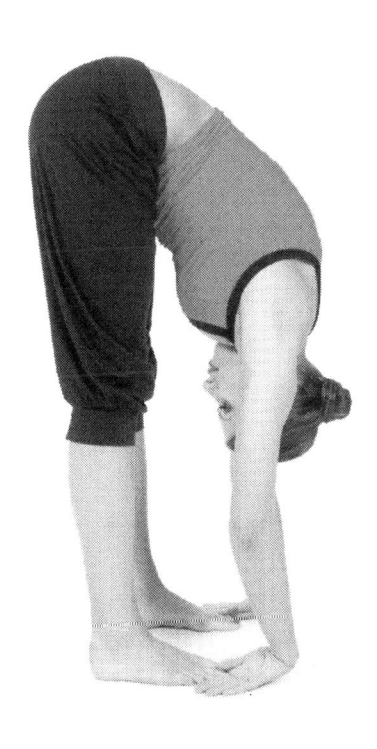

Instructions
1. Stand straight with your feet six inches apart.
2. Lift your kneecaps by contracting the thigh muscles.
3. Exhale, bending forward from the hips. As you bend, keep your head aligned with your torso.
4. Hold your big toes by sliding the index and middle fingers under the big toes and curling the fingers around them. Secure the fingers with the thumb.
5. Inhale. Lift your torso, still holding the big toes, and straighten your elbows.
6. Exhale as you lower your torso. Repeat this a few times, and with every time work towards extending the stretch.
7. After few repetitions, exhale and hold the position for one minute.
8. With inhalation lift your torso up, straighten your body, and bring your hands to your sides.

Note
If you find it difficult to reach your toes with your hands, use a strap or band to connect your hands with your feet.

Caution
Those with lower back pain or neck pain should not practice this pose.

Bharadvaja's Twist

Bharadvaja's twist is a pose named after Sage Bharadvaja.

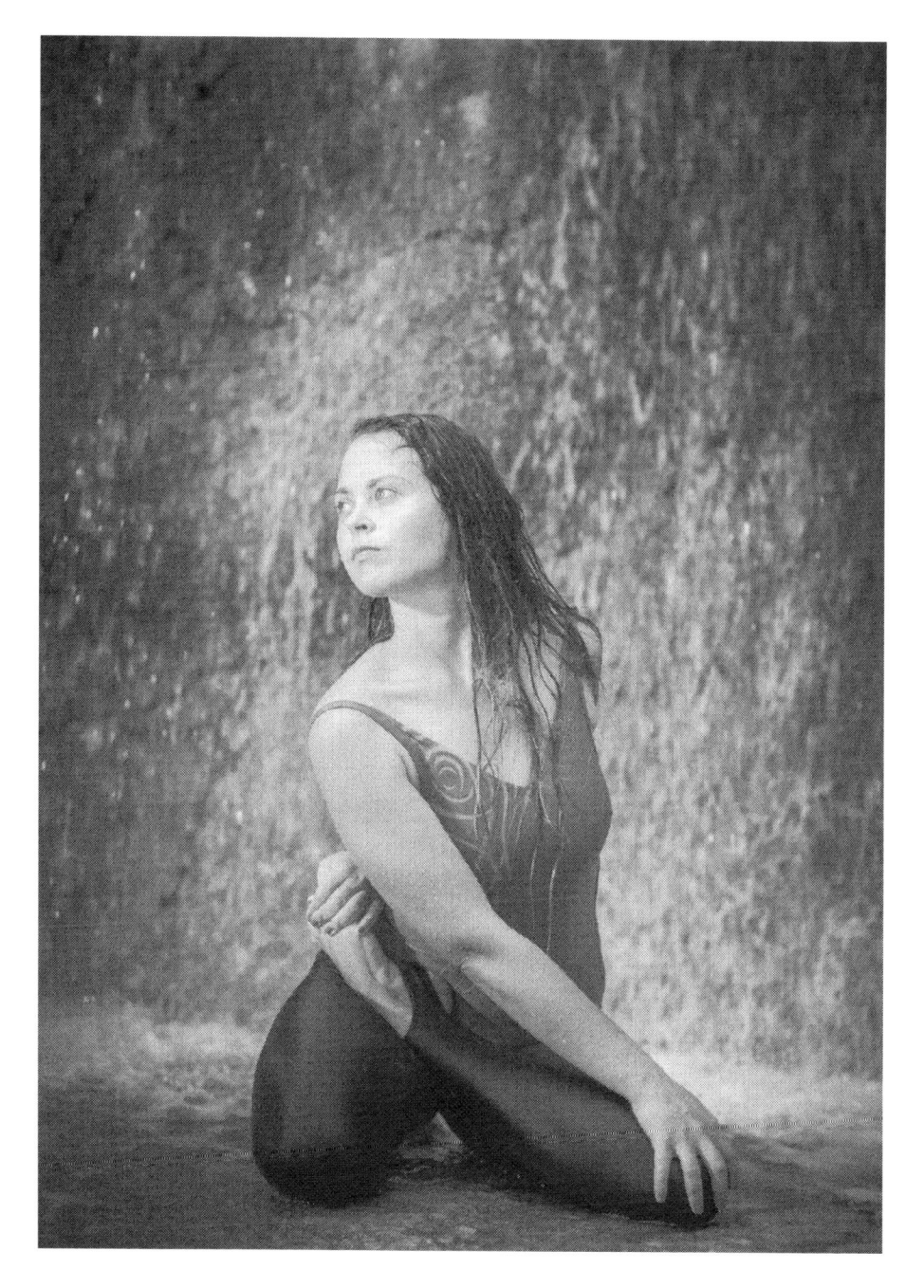

Instructions
1. Assume staff pose (p19).
2. Bend the right leg and place the lower leg by the outer side of the right thigh. Your heel should be close to the hips, as in hero pose.
3. Bend your left leg and place the left foot on top of the right thigh.
4. Twist your torso to your left.
5. Slide your left hand behind your back and hold the left foot.
6. Place your right hand on top of the left knee.
7. Turn your head towards the left, and look over the left shoulder. You can also close your eyes.
8. Remain in the pose for 30 seconds to one minute.
9. Repeat the same with the other leg.

Benefits
- Stretches and strengthens the shoulders
- Improves spine flexibility and tones the spine
- Relieves back pain
- Reduces sciatic pain
- Stimulates the function of the abdominal organs
- Improves digestion
- Offers some relief for carpal tunnel syndrome symptoms

Note
If keeping the knees down is difficult, place a folded blanket under your buttocks.

Caution
Those with high or low blood pressure or insomnia should avoid doing this pose. It is also not recommended to perform the pose while you have a headache, diarrhea, or during the menstrual cycle.

Cow Pose

Cow pose is sometimes integrated with cat pose, and together they form a short sequence.

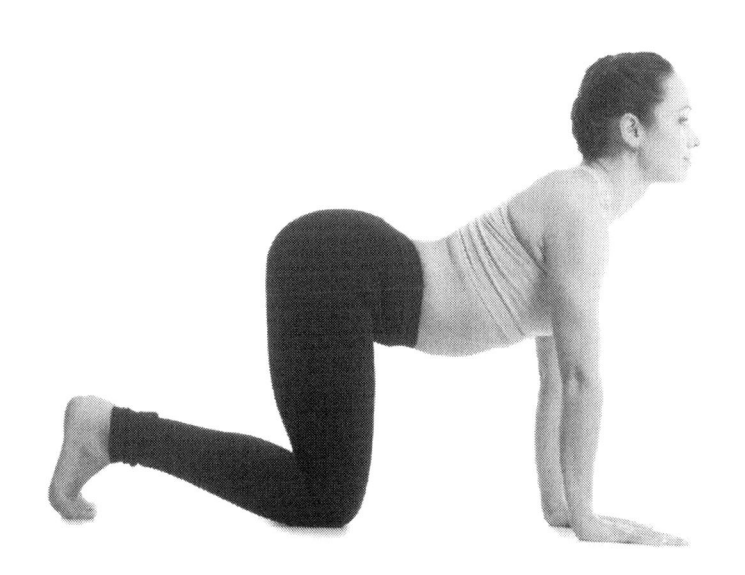

Instructions
1. Go on all fours by placing your palms and knees on the floor. Place your palms below your shoulders and your knees below your hips.
2. Keep your head in a neutral position, and look at the floor.
3. Inhale. Lift your butt and chest high as you gently push the belly downward.
4. Lift your head and look straight ahead.
5. Exhale, return to the initial position, and repeat the steps up to 20 times.

Benefits
- Stretches the spine, neck, and torso
- Boosts lung function
- Relieves muscular back pain

- Promotes shoulder flexibility
- Tones the back muscles
- Improves abdominal functions
- Corrects posture
- Promotes balance and a sense of calm

Note
You can keep the head straight if you have neck pain. If you have knee pain, place your knees on a folded blanket.

Caution
Those with a neck injury should not practice this pose.

Cat Pose

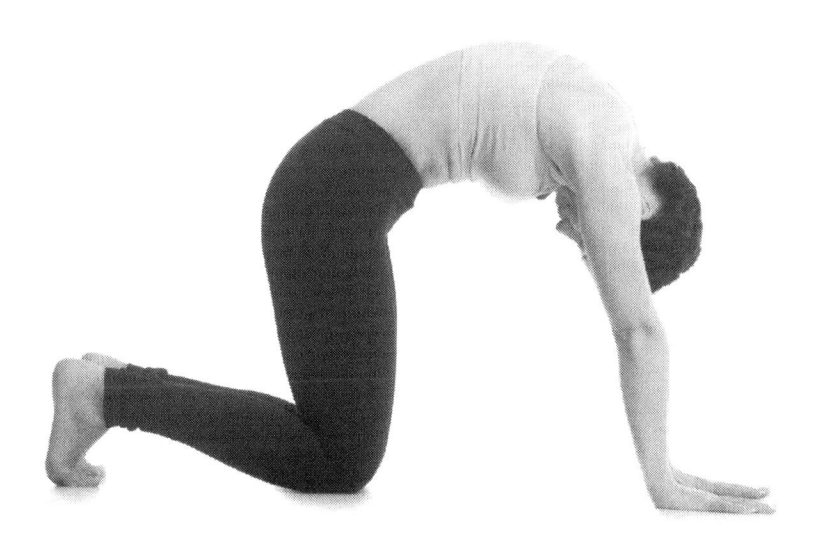

Instructions
1. Come down on all fours, positioning your knees and palms as in cow pose.
2. Keep your head in a neutral position.
3. With exhalation, lift your back as high as possible. The spine should be arched well. As you lift your back lower your chin, reaching for your chest. Your movements should be slow and gentle. Lower your chin to the extent you are comfortable.
4. Keep your buttocks relaxed.
5. Return to a tabletop position after a few seconds.
6. Repeat the steps up to 20 times.

Benefits
- Improves shoulder flexibility
- Strengthens the wrists
- Tones the spine and back
- Improves blood circulation

- Relieves back pain
- Stimulates functions of abdominal organs
- Relieves stress

Cat-cow Pose performed as a sequence tones your shoulders and back. Include cat-cow sequence in your yoga session for optimum results for shoulder and back pain.

Caution
Avoid performing the pose if you have a neck injury.

Bow Pose

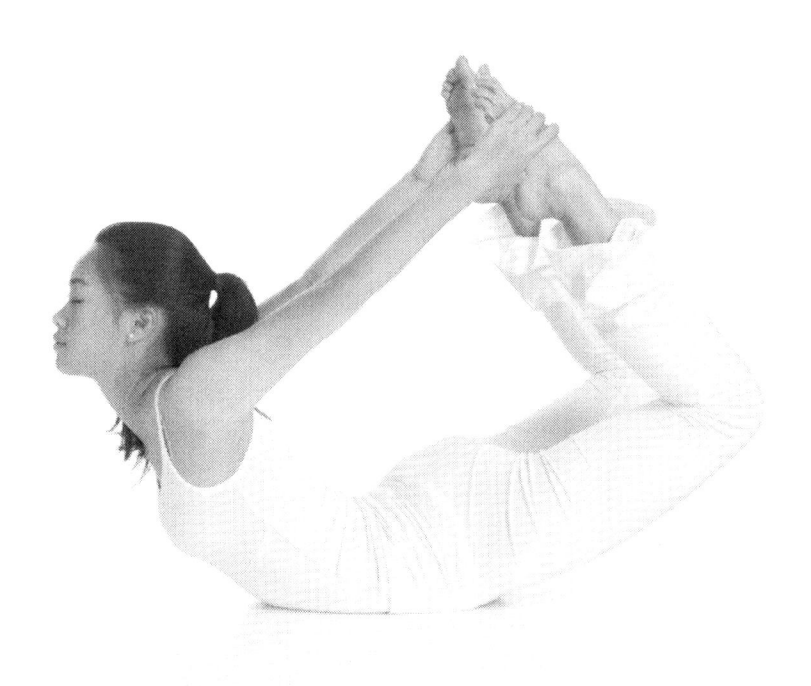

Instructions
1. Lie down on your stomach with your hands by your sides.
2. Bend your legs upwards, toward your head.
3. Stretch your hands back to hold the ankles.
4. With inhalation, lift your chest and thighs high so you are supported only by your abdomen. You will resemble a bow.
5. Remain in the pose for 20 seconds.
6. While coming out of the pose, place your torso and thighs on the mat, release your ankles, and place your hands and legs on the floor.

Benefits
- Stretches the entire front side of the body from the neck to the ankles
- Opens the shoulders, chest, and hips
- Strengthens the shoulders and improves shoulder flexibility
- Tones the spine and strengthens the back muscles
- Improves respiratory functions
- Reduces tummy fat
- Relieves constipation
- Improves digestion
- Boosts blood circulation
- Helps with menstrual disorders
- Stimulates the kidneys, liver, and pancreas

Note
A yoga strap can be used to hold the legs if it is difficult for you to reach your ankles with your hands. You can also place a folded blanket or yoga blocks under your thighs to help you pull them up.

Caution
Those with high or low blood pressure, neck or back injury, or hernia should not perform this pose. Do not perform this pose if you have a headache.

Camel Pose

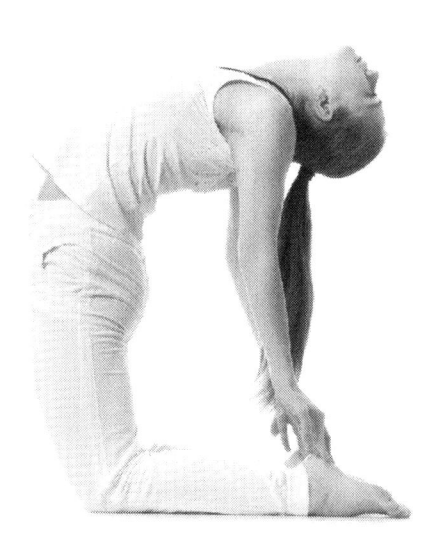

Instructions
1. Kneel on the mat with your legs hip-width apart
2. Place your hands behind your hips. The tops of your feet should be on the floor.
3. Bend back, and bring your hands down to hold the ankles.
4. Keep the thighs straight, so your hips are aligned with your knees and your back gets a good arch.
5. Lift your chin up so you face the wall behind you.
6. Remain in the pose for 30 seconds.
7. Come out of the pose by first releasing your hands and then straightening your back.

Benefits
- Stretches the front of the body from the chest to the thighs
- Tones the spine and increases spine flexibility
- Strengthens the back muscles
- Energizes the whole body
- Strengthens the shoulders and improves their flexibility

- Improves lung function and aids in curing respiratory conditions, including asthma
- Stimulates the functions of the abdominal organs
- Improves posture

Note

Tuck in your toes and raise your heels to hold them if you are unable to reach for your ankles. Alternately, you can place a block under your feet to increase the height so holding the ankles will be easier. You can also place your hands behind your hips if you are unable to hold your ankles.

Caution

Those with high or low blood pressure or back conditions should refrain from practicing this pose.

Intermediate Poses for Strengthening the Shoulders

Side Plank Pose

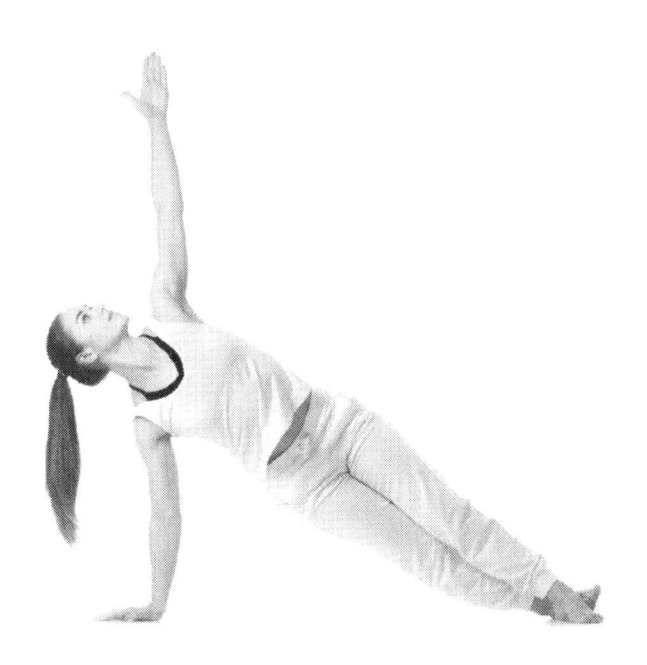

Instructions
1. Go into downward facing dog pose, in which your palms and feet are on the ground and your hips are high, so you resemble an inverted 'V.'
2. Lower your hips, as in plank pose.
3. Twist your legs to your right, so the outer edge of your right foot is on the floor and the left foot is beside the right.
4. With your right hand firmly on the ground, roll over to your right.
5. Lift the left arm off the ground and stretch it towards the ceiling.

6. Your shoulders should be aligned, and your body in one straight line.
7. Fix your gaze at the top of the thumb of your extended hand.
8. Remain in the pose for 30 seconds.
9. Repeat the same steps on the other side.

Benefits
- Strengthens the shoulders, arms, and wrists
- Strengthens your spine and tones your back
- Stretches the back of the thighs and the calf muscles
- Strengthens the body core
- Tones the abdominal muscles
- Improves balance
- Improves focus

Note
Beginners can place the knee of the bottom leg on the floor for support.

Caution
Do not practice the pose if you have any injury to your shoulders, arms, wrists, or back.

Eagle Pose

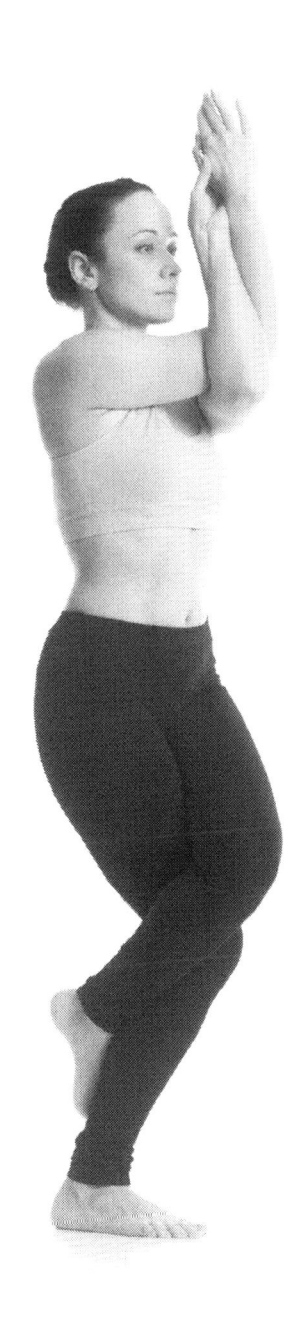

Instructions
1. Stand straight with your hands by your sides.
2. Bend your knees and curl the left leg around the right leg, so the left thigh rests on the right thigh and the left foot will be behind the right calf muscle.
3. Stretch your arms in front of your body. Bring the left hand under the right.
4. Bend your elbows, and curl the forearms so the palms face each other and the forearms are entwined.
5. Lift your elbows so the forearms are perpendicular to the ground, with your fingers pointed upwards.
6. Remain in the pose for 30 seconds.
7. Come out of the pose by uncurling your hands and then legs.
8. Repeat the same steps on the other side.

Benefits
- Stretches the shoulders, arms, and upper back
- Strengthens the leg muscles and ankles
- Strengthens the hips
- Boosts lung capacity and relieves respiratory disorders
- Relieves lower back pain
- Relieves sciatic pain
- Improves flexibility of the joints
- Corrects posture
- Improves focus
- Promotes balance

Note
Those with low blood pressure or ear problems impairing the balance can practice this pose against the wall.

Caution
Those with a severe knee, ankle, or hip injury should refrain from practicing the pose.

Basic Poses for Strengthening the Core

Strengthening your core balances your body. If your core is strong, your level of stability will be good and so will your posture. You will love the fact that your tummy becomes flat and strong when your core is strengthened. Core strength also improves coordination and reduces the risk of injury. It improves your flexibility and relieves back pain, which is one of the most common health issues faced by the world population, mainly those who do desk work.

What is the core? The core is the torso of your body, and all the muscles in the front, back, and the sides of your midsection.

Yoga helps to strengthen your core and minimizes the risk of all injuries and conditions caused due to weakness in this area. Certain yoga poses target the muscle groups here and strengthen them, thereby aiding in overall health.

While there are tougher poses for core strength, beginners can start with the ones mentioned here, which are effective for developing core strength.

Boat Pose

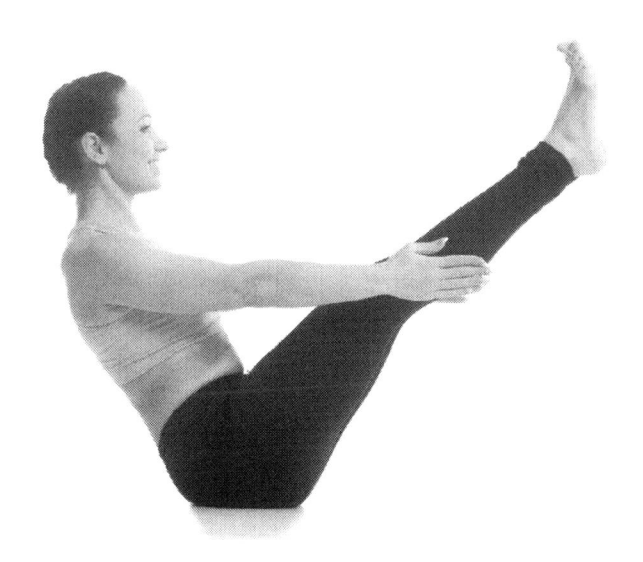

Instructions

1. Sit down with your knees bent and your feet on the ground. Keep the hands by the sides of your hips.
2. Lean back a bit with your spine erect.
3. Lift your feet off the floor and straighten your legs.
4. Extend your arms so they are in a straight line with your shoulders.
5. With your spine and legs straight, balance on your sit bones. You should be in a 'V' shape.
6. Keep your face straight ahead, and breathe normally.
7. Remain in the pose for 30 seconds to one minute.

Benefits

- Strengthens abdominal muscles, reduces tummy fat
- Improves core strength
- Strengthens the lower back
- Stimulates the abdominal organs and optimizes their function

- Maintains a healthy metabolism
- Relieves indigestion
- Regulates thyroid function
- Relieves stress

Note
If lifting the legs is difficult, you can use a strap looped around your feet. Holding the strap, you can straighten your legs.

Alternatively, you may place a block under your feet. However, to aid in perfecting the pose, it is recommended to maintain very light contact with the block, instead of placing your feet on it.

Caution
Those with insomnia should refrain from practicing this pose. Those with asthma and heart conditions can perform one of the gentler versions. If you have neck or back injuries, lean against a wall for practicing this pose. Do not perform the pose when you have a headache, diarrhea, low blood pressure, or during menstruation.

Locust Pose

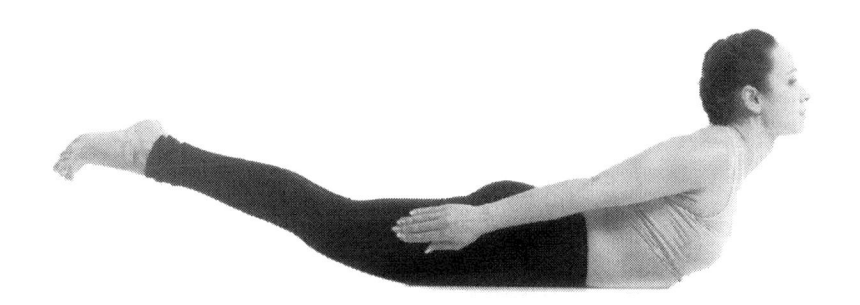

Instructions
1. Lie down on your stomach, placing the legs together. Rest your hands by your sides.
2. Rest your chin on the floor. Inhale.
3. Pressing the pubic bone firmly on the ground, lift your legs, arms, chin, and chest off the ground.
4. Your arms should be parallel to the ground and stretched backwards.
5. You will now be resting on your belly, front pelvis, and lower ribs.
6. Look straight ahead or slightly lift your chin upward.
7. Remain in the pose for one minute.

Benefits
- Strengthens the core, shoulders, and arms
- Opens the chest
- Improves spine flexibility
- Relieves constipation
- Improves digestion

Note

If lifting the upper torso and thighs is difficult, place a rolled blanket under your ribcage and another under your thighs.

Caution

Avoid performing this pose if you have a back injury. Lotus pose is also not recommended for those with severe injury in the shoulders or arms. Do not practice the pose during menstruation.

Half Prayer Twist

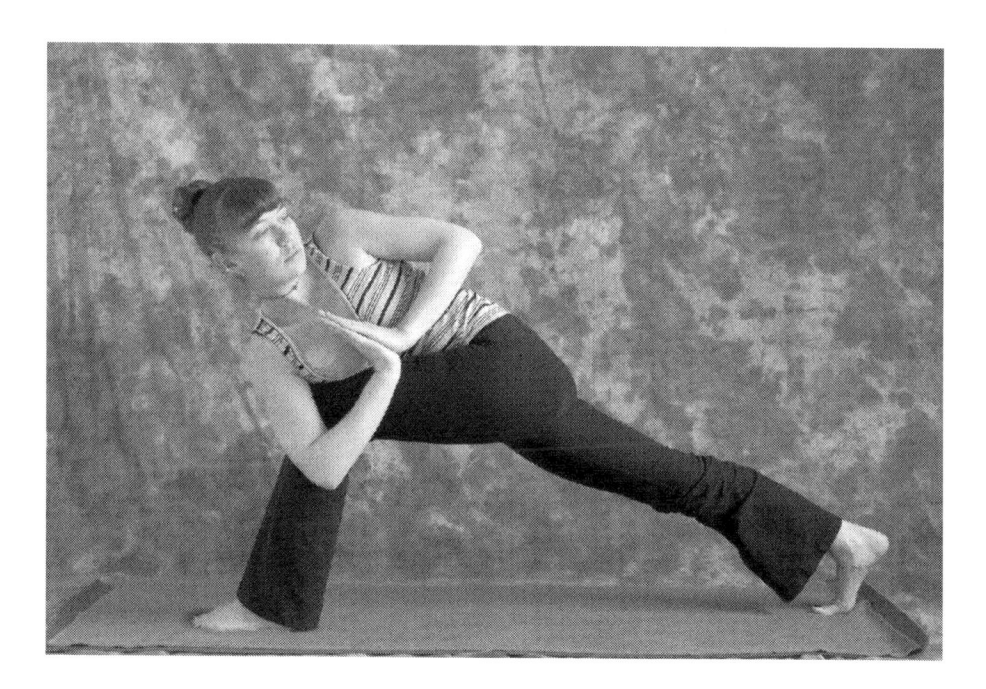

Instructions
1. Go into table pose, in which you are on all fours with your palms, knees, and toes on the floor.
2. Bring your right leg forward and place the right foot between your hands. Your right knee should be aligned with your right ankle.
3. Twist your torso to the right and place the left elbow on the outer side of your right knee. Bring your palms together in front of your chest in prayer pose. Your fingers should be pointing at your throat.
4. Twist your upper back as much as you can, so the right shoulder is raised and stretched.
5. Remain in the pose for 30 seconds.
6. To come out of the pose, exhale as you bring the arms to the floor. Stretch your front leg back as in table pose, and sit down.
7. Repeat the same steps on the other side.

Benefits
- Tones the core
- Opens the chest and hips
- Stretches the spine and tones the back

Caution

Those with an injury to the shoulders, back, or hips should avoid practicing this pose.

Dolphin Pose

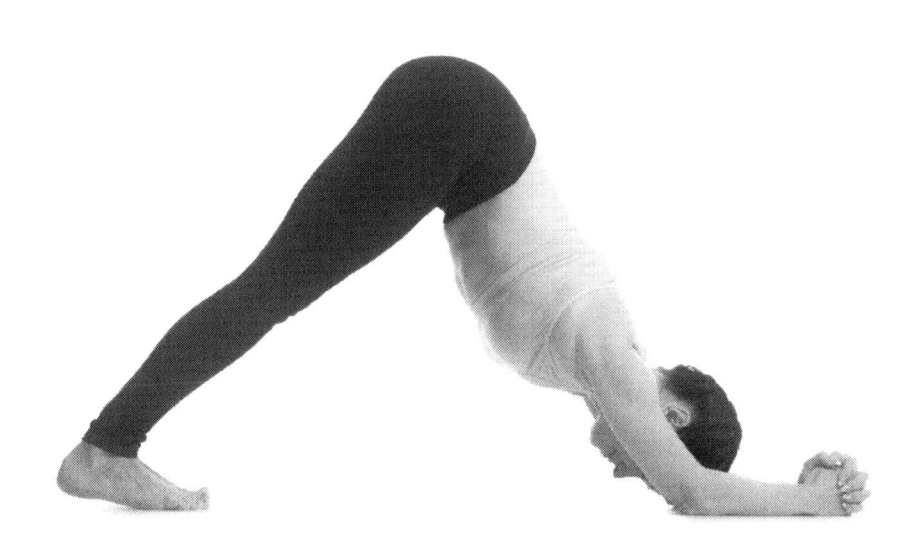

Instructions

1. Go down on all fours with your hands and knees on the ground. Your arms should be perpendicular to the floor, and your knees aligned with your hips.
2. Lower your elbows to place your forearms on the floor in front of your knees. Your hands and forearms should be straight and parallel to each other.
3. Tuck your toes in, and lift your knees away from the ground.
4. Lift your sitting bones high towards the ceiling as you straighten your knees.
5. Let your head be held between you forearms.
6. Now you will resemble an inverted 'V'.
7. Remain in the pose for 30 seconds to one minute.
8. To come out of the pose, place your knees on the floor, and relax.

Benefits
- Strengthens the core, arms, and legs
- Stretches the shoulders, hips, and legs
- Energizes the body
- Promotes respiratory function
- Improves digestion
- Tones the back muscles and relieves back pain
- Relieves menstrual discomfort and menopausal symptoms
- Lowers high blood pressure
- Relieves sciatic pain
- Prevents osteoporosis
- Cures headache
- Improves flat feet
- Relieves mild depression
- Boosts memory

Note
Beginners can place a folded blanket under the elbows to gain some height to support lifting.

Caution
Those with injury in the shoulders, neck, arms, or back should not practice this pose. This pose is also not recommended for those with high blood pressure, or infection in the eye or ear.

One-Legged Down Dog Pose

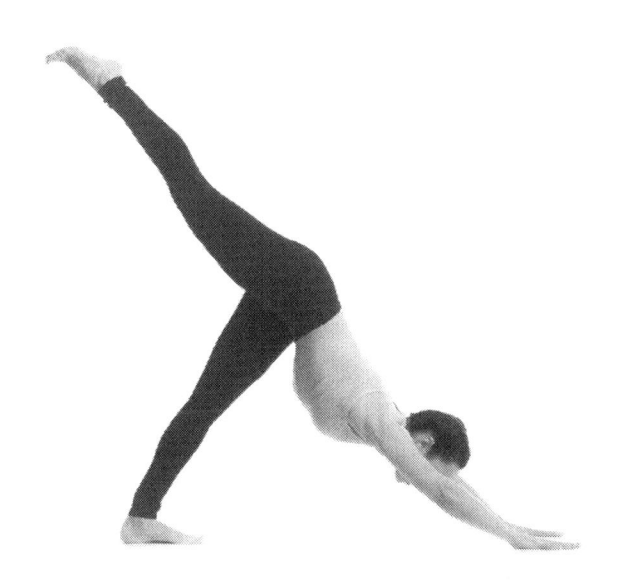

Instructions
1. Begin in downward facing dog pose.
2. Lift the right leg off the floor and stretch it as high as possible.
3. The toes of the right leg should be pointed towards the ground.
4. The extended right leg should be in line with your body.
5. Square your hips and shoulders.
6. Remain in the pose for one minute.
7. Repeat the same steps with the other leg.

Benefits
- Strengthens the arms and legs
- Strengthens the core
- Improves spine flexibility
- Promotes blood flow
- Improves balance
- Calms the mind

Caution
Avoid practicing this pose if you have high blood pressure, carpal tunnel syndrome, or injury in your shoulders, wrists, or ankles.

Extended Triangle Pose

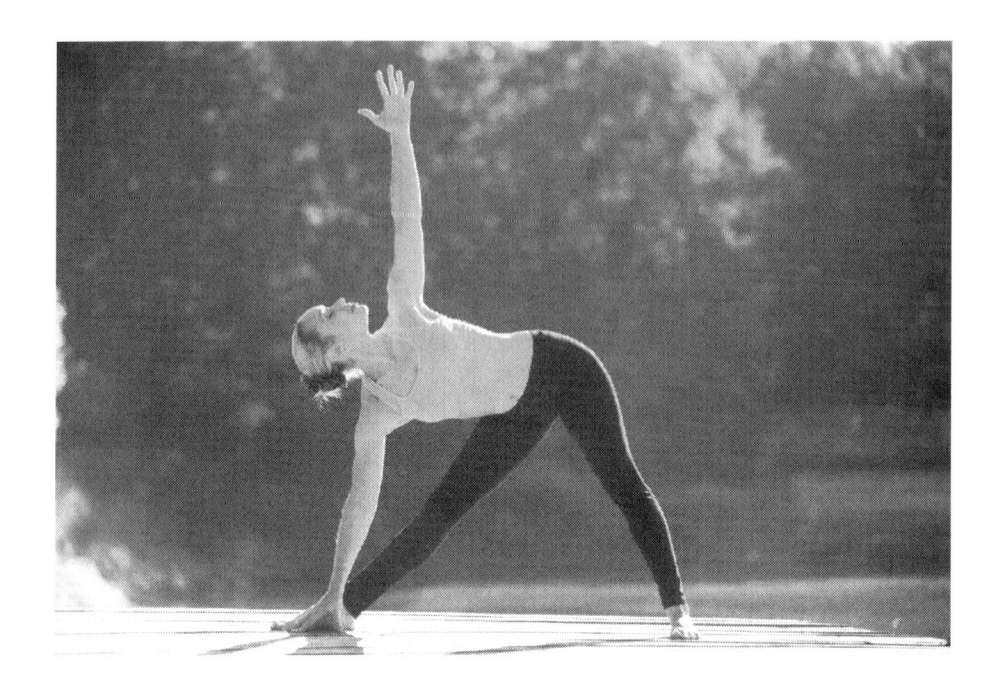

Instructions
1. Stand straight with your hands by your sides.
2. Exhale, and step your left foot back, maintaining a distance of about three to four feet.
3. Turn the left foot in slightly so the heels are in line.
4. Inhale and lift your hands to shoulder level, keeping the elbows straight and the hands parallel to the ground. Now your hands and shoulders are in a straight line.
5. Bend at the right side to bring the right hand down.
6. Place the right palm on the outer side of the right foot. Do not lean forward. Your hips should be straight.
7. Stretch your left hand up towards the ceiling.
8. Turn your head up and gaze at the fingers of the extended hand. You can also look straight ahead.
9. Remain in the pose for one minute.
10. Repeat the same with the other leg.

Benefits
- Stretches the shoulders, groin, hips, and legs
- Stretches and strengthens the spine
- Strengthens the core
- Boosts energy
- Tones the back muscles
- Relieves back pain
- Stimulates the abdominal organs
- Improves digestion
- Relieves stress
- Promotes balance

Note

Do not push hard if your hand does not reach the ground. Use a block to place your palm on.

Caution

If you have neck pain, you can keep your head straight instead of turning upwards. Those with high blood pressure should turn their head downwards. Avoid practicing the pose if you have low blood pressure. Do not practice the pose when you are experiencing headache or diarrhea.

Other beginner yoga poses for strengthening the core include:
- Reverse Table Top Pose (p69)
- Plank Pose (p73)
- Chair Pose (p82)

Intermediate Poses for Strengthening the Core

Tiptoe Pose

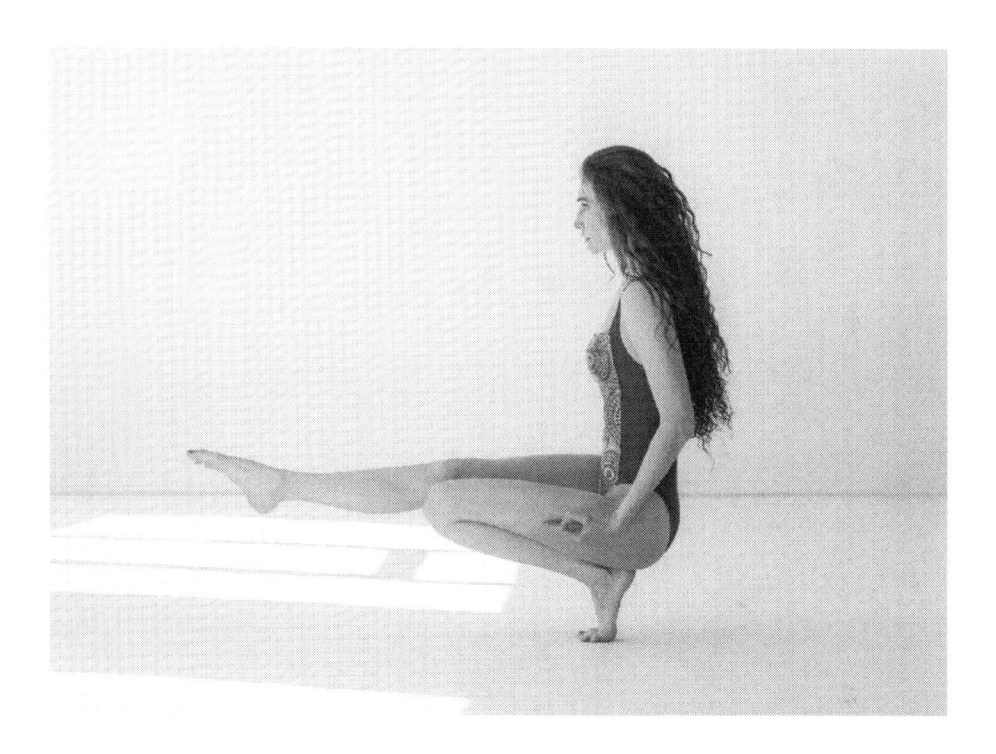

Instructions
1. Stand straight, and exhale as you lower your body towards the floor.
2. Lift your heels off the ground so your weight is balanced on your toes.
3. Sit on your heels, and keep your back straight.
4. Place your palms together in front of your chest.
5. Fix your focus at the center of your eyebrows.
6. Remain in the pose for 30 seconds.

More challenging variation of this pose:

1. Lower the arms to the side of the thighs, bring the tips of your index finger and thumb together in slight contact.
2. For more of a challenge, stretch a leg straight in front of you.
3. Remain in the pose for 30 seconds.
4. Release the pose by placing your heels down. Lift your torso and stand straight.

Benefits
- Strengthens the core
- Strengthens the entire leg
- Improves the flexibility of the legs
- Stretches and strengthens the hips
- Tones the abdominal muscles
- Supports the reproductive system
- Promotes balance

Caution
Those with hip injury, or back or knee problems should refrain from practicing this pose.

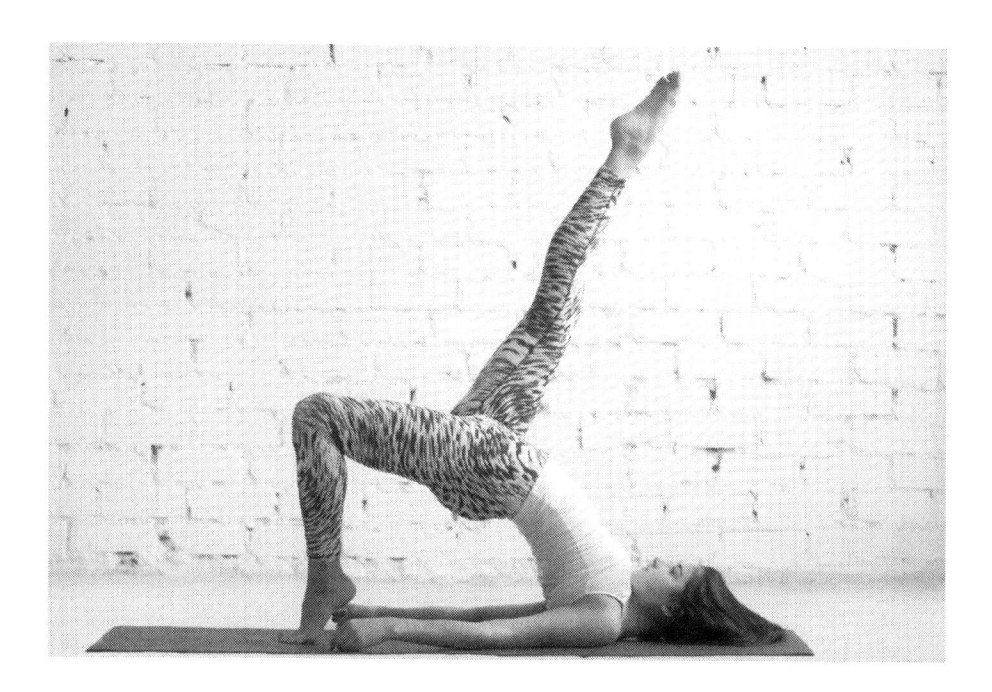

One-Legged Bridge Pose

Instructions
1. Lie down on your back, keeping the knees bent and your hands by your sides. Your knees should be directly over your ankles.
2. Pressing the arms and feet firmly on the floor, raise your hips.
3. Slide your hands under your body and interlock your fingers.
4. Pressing the left foot firmly down, bend your right leg and bring the right knee forward.
5. Stretch the right leg up until the leg is vertical to the ground.
6. Lengthen your spine and lift your hips higher.
7. Remain in the pose for 30 seconds.
8. To come out of the pose, return the right leg to the floor, stretch your legs, release your hands, and bring them to the sides.
9. Repeat the same steps on the other side.

Benefits
- Strengthens the core
- Strengthens the shoulders, arms, and legs
- Expands the chest, and relieves respiratory conditions
- Stretches the spine, neck, and thighs
- Stimulates the function of the abdominal organs
- Improves digestion
- Relieves insomnia
- Regulates thyroid function
- Builds strength
- Relieves stress
- Cures mild depression

Note
Beginners can keep their hands by their sides instead of clasping them behind the back. The hands can also be placed under the hips to hold the hips higher.

Caution
Those with shoulder, neck, or hip injuries should not perform this pose.

Four-Limbed Staff Pose

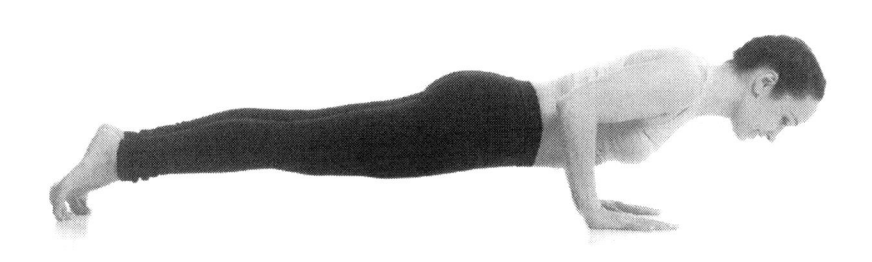

Instructions
1. Start with plank pose, in which your palms and feet are on the floor, with your hands and legs fully stretched and your back flat.
2. Rock a little forward and keep your elbows close to your body.
3. Exhale, while lowering your body towards the floor until your upper arms are parallel to the ground.
4. Roll out the shoulders.
5. Remain in the pose for 30 seconds.
6. To release the pose, inhale and move to upward facing dog pose (p77). Release down.

Benefits
- Strengthens the core
- Strengthens the shoulders, arms, and wrists
- Improves stability
- Strengthens the back
- Tones the entire body

Note
Beginners can keep their knees on the ground for support, and drop the torso lower. With practice, the body will become stronger and the pose can be mastered.

Caution
Those with carpal tunnel syndrome should not practice this pose. Those with injury to the shoulders, elbows, and wrists should also avoid practicing this pose.

Basic Poses for the Hips

Tight hips can be very uncomfortable, as they compromise your flexibility. Tight hips mean the spine has to work harder, so releasing that tension in your hips increases your overall flexibility and wellbeing. To lessen the impact of a sedentary lifestyle on your mobility, it is essential that hip opening poses are performed regularly. It's also said that hip opening poses unlock your creativity.

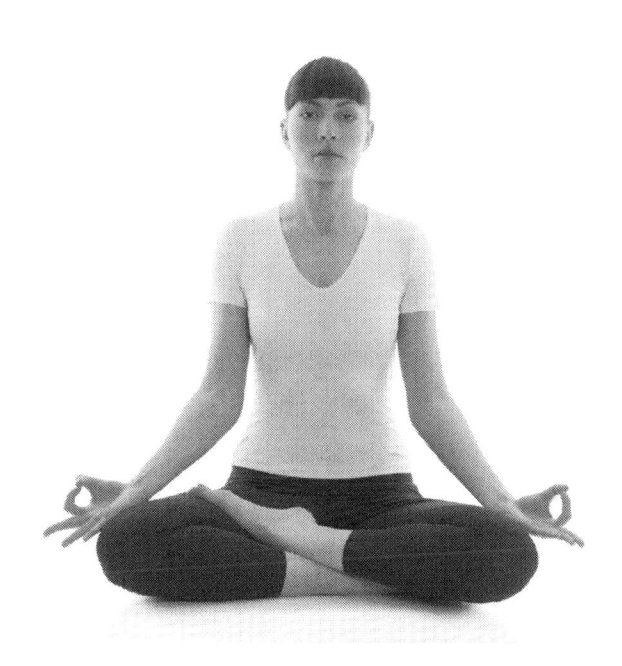

Easy Pose

Instructions
1. Sit on the mat, keeping your legs stretched out and your back straight.
2. Bend your right leg. Hold your right foot and place it below the left thigh.

3. Similarly, bend your left leg, hold your left foot, and place it below the right thigh.
4. Keep the spine erect.
5. Place your palms on your knees. Perform chin mudra (bringing your thumb and index fingers together in light contact and the other three fingers stretched).
6. Remain in the pose for one minute, initially. With practice you can increase the duration up to one hour, as this pose is recommended for meditation.

Benefits
- Strengthens the spine
- Tones the back muscles
- Opens the hips and angles
- Stretches the knees and ankles
- Relieves stress
- Calms the mind

Caution
Those with a knee injury should refrain from practicing this pose.

Half Lord of the Fishes Pose

Also called half spinal twist, half lord of the fishes pose is an advanced version of twisted pose (but still a basic pose).

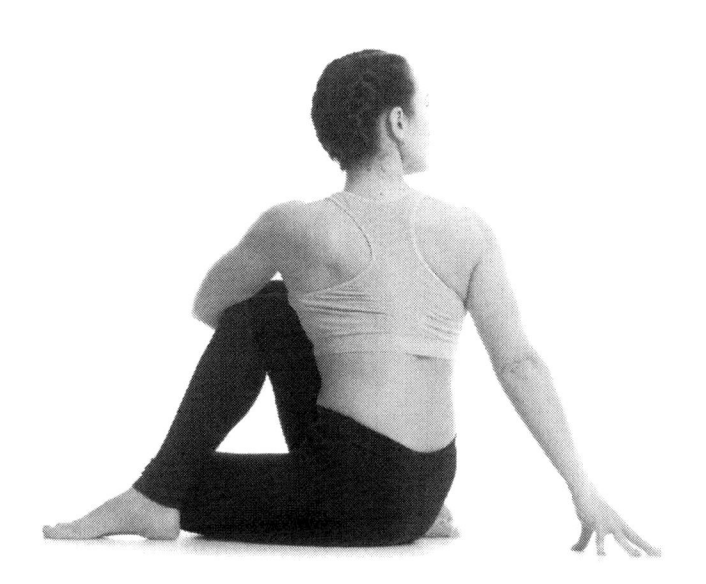

Instructions
1. Sit down. Stretch your legs forward.
2. Bend your left leg and bring the left foot over the extended right leg, and place it on the floor adjacent to the outer right hip.
3. Slide your right leg on the floor, bringing the right heel towards you and placing it near the left buttock.
4. Twist your torso towards your left.
5. Place your left hand behind your back on the floor. If you stretch further, you can slide your left hand behind your back to hold the left ankle.
6. Bring your right hand over the left leg, and place your palm on the right knee.
7. Turn your head to look over your left shoulder. Those with discomfort when turning the head can look straight.

8. Remain in the pose for 30 seconds to one minute.
9. Return to basic position, and repeat the same steps on the other side.

Benefits
- Makes the spine flexible
- Strengthens the nervous system
- Reduces fat in the midsection
- Tones the back muscles and relieves back pain
- Relieves the symptoms of asthma
- Cures menstrual discomfort
- Promotes blood flow in the pelvic region
- Improves fertility
- Boosts liver and kidney functions
- Relieves fatigue
- Awakens Kundalini power, an energy that lies dormant in Muladhara

Caution
Those with back injuries or spinal problems should not practice this pose. Beginners are requested to attempt the pose without pushing beyond the limit of their own comfort.

Child's Pose

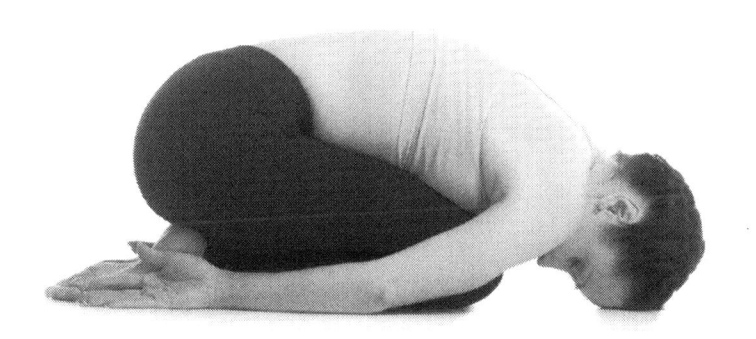

Instructions
1. Kneel down with your thighs together.
2. Bring your big toes together, and keep the heels apart. This will make your feet look like a 'V'.
3. Sit down on the space between your heels, and keep your back straight.
4. Inhale and lift your hands over your head.
5. Exhale as you bend forward with your hands stretched upwards.
6. Place your hands on the ground, stretching the arms well. Alternately, you can place your hands by your sides with palms turned upwards.
7. Lengthen your spine and place your forehead on the ground in front of your knees. Do not lift the buttocks.
8. Remain in the pose for one minute.
9. Inhale as you come out of the pose.

Benefits
- Stretches and strengthens your spine
- Tones your back muscles
- Opens the hips
- Relaxes the neck and shoulders
- Calms the nervous system
- Improves digestion
- Relieves constipation
- Promotes blood flow to the head
- Calms the mind

Caution

Those with high blood pressure or knee injuries should refrain from practicing this pose.

Bound Angle Pose

Also called cobbler's pose, bound angle pose is one of the best hip-openers for beginners.

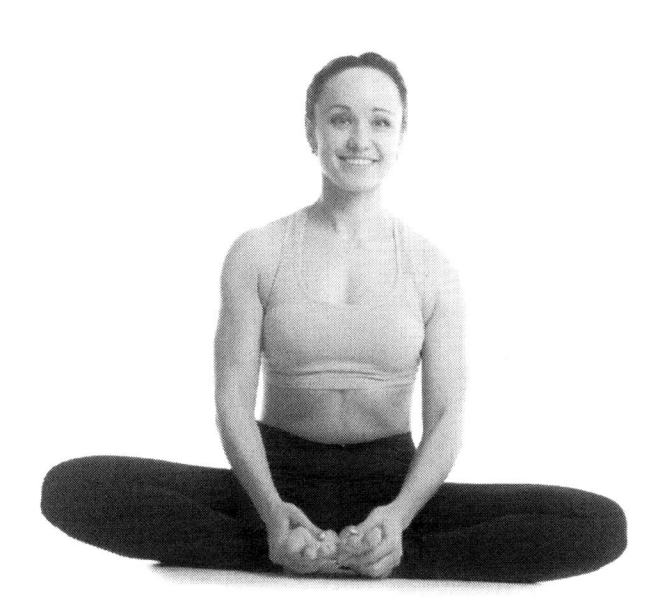

Instructions
1. Sit down with your spine erect and your legs extended in front of you.
2. Bend your knees and bring the heels close to your pelvis.
3. Place the soles of your feet together.
4. Hold the big toes with your index and middle fingers, secured with the thumb.
5. Lengthen the spine.
6. Look straight ahead.
7. Remain in the pose for three to five minutes.

Benefits
- Stretches the hips
- Tones the thighs
- Tones the heart
- Stimulates the abdominal organs
- Lowers high blood pressure
- Promotes blood flow throughout the body
- Improves fertility
- Relieves menstrual discomfort
- Relieves sciatic pain
- Works for flat feet
- Supports easy childbirth
- Relieves stress and fatigue
- Promotes calm

Caution
Do not practice the pose if you have an injury in your knees or groin.

Reclining Bound Angle Pose

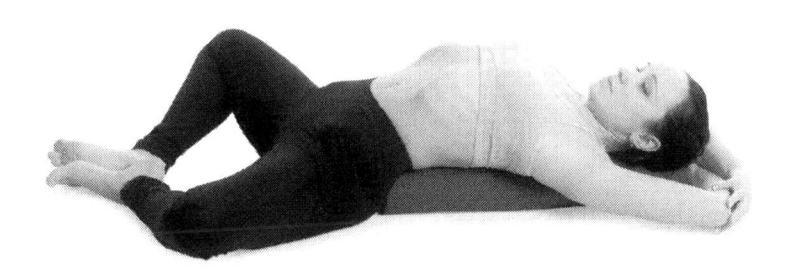

Instructions
1. Perform bound angle pose.
2. Lean back and place your elbows on the ground.
3. Gently lower the body and lie down on your back.
4. Relax your back, shoulders, and arms.
5. Keep your arms slightly away from your body.
6. Close your eyes.
7. Remain in the pose for one minute. As you progress, you can increase the duration up to 10 minutes.
8. Bring your knees together. Turn to your right. Place the left hand on the floor, press, and get up.

Benefits
- Opens the hips
- Calms the nerves
- Opens the chest
- Improves respiratory function
- Boosts energy
- Lowers high blood pressure
- Relieves muscular tension
- Cures fatigue
- Relieves stress

Cow Face Pose

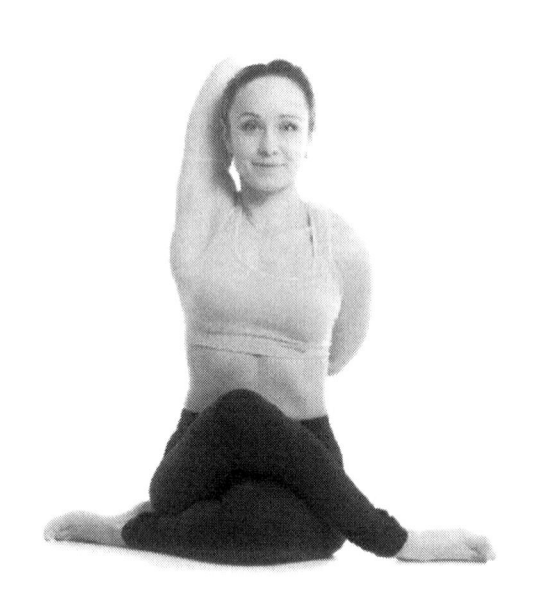

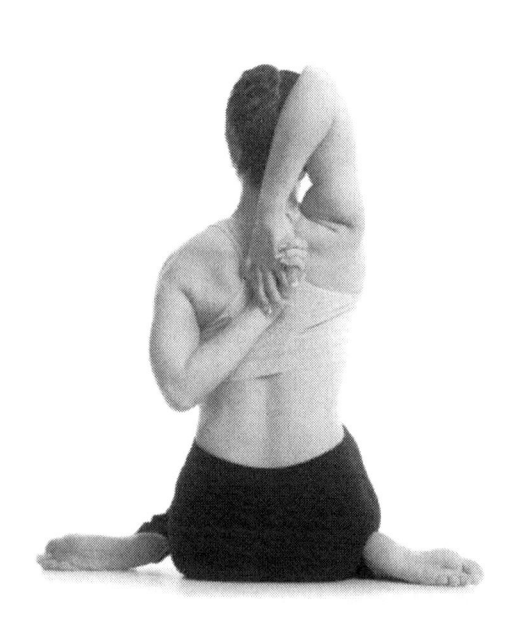

Instructions
1. Sit straight with your legs stretched in front of you.
2. Bend your left leg and slide the left foot under the right thigh. Place the foot on the outer side of the right hip. The left heel should be closer to the buttocks.
3. Place your right leg over the left and draw the right foot beyond the left hip. The right knee should be over the left knee.
4. Sit on your sitting bones with your weight evenly spread.
5. With inhalation, extend your right arm parallel to the ground, thumb down, so that the palm faces backward.
6. Slide your right hand behind your torso and bring the right palm up towards your shoulder blade. Your right elbow should near your torso.
7. Inhale, and stretch your left hand upwards, turn your palm up and raise the hand towards the ceiling.
8. Bend your left elbow and bring the hand over your shoulders. Lock the fingers of your hands together.
9. Hold the pose for one minute.
10. Repeat the same with the other hand and leg.

Note
If you are unable to stretch until your hands come together, use yoga strap and hold it at the ends.

Caution
Those with severe neck or shoulder problems should avoid practicing this pose.

Other poses for opening the hips include:
- Bharadvaja's Twist (p. 109)

Intermediate Poses for the Hips

Half Pigeon Pose

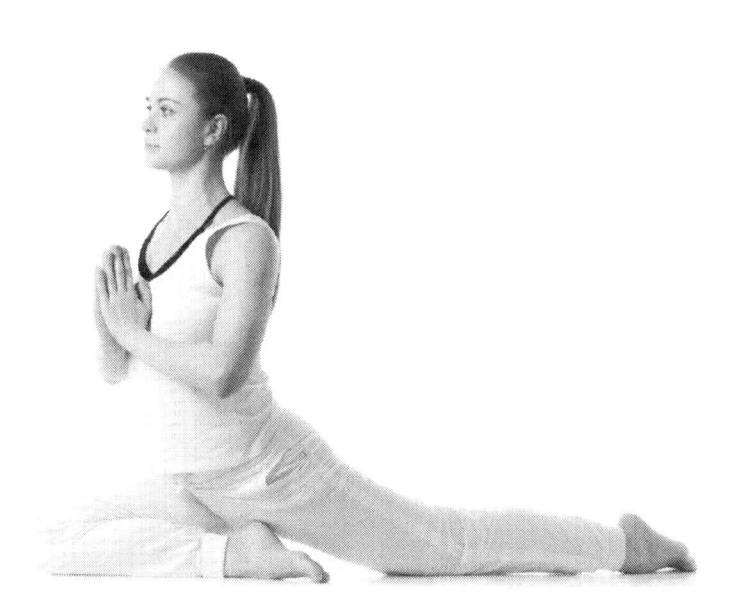

Instructions
1. Go on your knees, and sit on your heels.
2. Lean forward and place your palms in front of you on the floor. They should be shoulder-width apart.
3. Lift yourself so you are on all fours. Your knees should be shoulder-width apart.
4. Draw your body forward, bending your right leg so the shin and the back of the thigh are on the floor. Your right knee should be aligned with your right hip and your foot should be facing down.
5. Stretch your left leg backwards, keeping the top of foot on the floor.
6. Lengthen your spine and lift your torso. Square your hips so your upper body is facing frontwards.
7. Balance your body weight evenly between your hips.

8. Fix your gaze downwards, and place your hands in a praying position.
9. Remain in the pose for one minute.
10. To come out of the pose, tuck your toes of the back leg in, lift the knee, and transition to downward facing dog pose.
11. Repeat the same steps on the other side.

Benefits
- Opens the hips and improves hip flexibility
- Stretches and strengthens the legs
- Expands the chest and improves respiratory conditions
- Stretches the neck and shoulders
- Stretches the spine and improves its flexibility
- Boosts blood circulation
- Tones the abdominal organs and improves their performance

Note
If you have difficulty in placing the thigh of the bent leg on the floor, place a folded blanket under it for support.

Do not attempt the pose beyond the limit of your comfort. Listen to your body and practice only as much as your body allows. With practice you will be able to perform the pose to perfection.

Caution
Do not perform the pose if you have a hip or knee injury.

Extended Hand-To-Big-Toe Pose

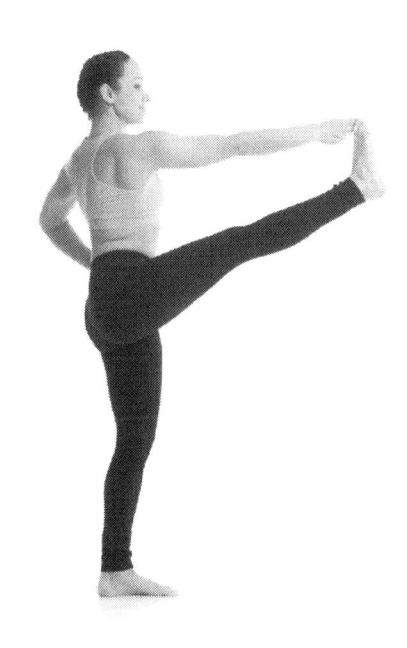

Instructions
1. Stand straight, placing your feet together. Keep your arms by your sides.
2. With the left foot firmly on the ground, draw your right knee towards your chest.
3. Bring your right arm from your side to the inner side of your right thigh.
4. Encircle your right big toe with your index and middle fingers.
5. Bend your left arm and hold the left hip.
6. Lengthen your spine.
7. Exhale as you stretch your right leg forward, supported by your right hand. Stretch the leg as much as possible.
8. Square your hips and stretch your shoulders and neck.
9. Remain in the pose for 30 seconds.

10. To come out of the pose, bring your right knee closer to your chest, release your toes, and place the foot on the floor.
11. Repeat the same steps on the other side.

Benefits
- Opens the hips
- Stretches and strengthens the leg muscles and ankles
- Stretches the shoulders and arms
- Stabilizes the core
- Promotes good balance
- Improves focus
- Calms the mind

Note
You can use a support under the foot of extended leg. If you have difficulty in stretching the lifted leg, perform the pose with yoga strap, which is wrapped around your foot and held in the corresponding hand.

Caution
Those with a lower back injury or ankle injury should refrain from practicing this pose.

Yoga for Various Health Conditions

Yoga cures, or contributes to the reduction in symptoms of various health conditions. Yoga stimulates the function of all the systems of your body, from the circulatory system to the skeletal system and the endocrine system. It regulates the functions of organs and glands and works as a preventive exercise.

Yoga attempts to address the root of any ailment, and help the body heal itself. It improves the functions of organs affected by health issues, thereby aiding the body in its process of healing.

Regular practice of yoga encourages healthy eating habits, and enhances your lifestyle by improving your preferences for healthy ways like balanced eating, avoiding junk foods, getting a good sleep, and practicing yoga regularly. The better your choices are, higher the quality of your life will be.

As you well know, negativity in your mind affects your body, and disease in your body affects your mind. Yoga has the power to calm your mind, relieve negative emotions, and help you develop a positive attitude towards life. You learn acceptance, which goes a long way in keeping you physically and mentally healthy.

In the following pages, you will find yoga poses aimed at supporting your body through various diseases. Practicing the poses will help relieve your symptoms, and aid in healing.

Yoga for Headache

Headaches are caused by various factors including indigestion, neck pain, poor circulation, colds and sinus infections, eye strain and vision problems, hormonal fluctuations, postural problems, physical and mental stress, and sleeplessness. Yoga addresses many of these causes. It improves blood and oxygen flow, aids digestion, and stretches the body. It also relieves stress, a common cause of headache, and relaxes the mind. Regular practice of yoga reduces the occurrence of headaches and promotes overall health.

Lotus Pose

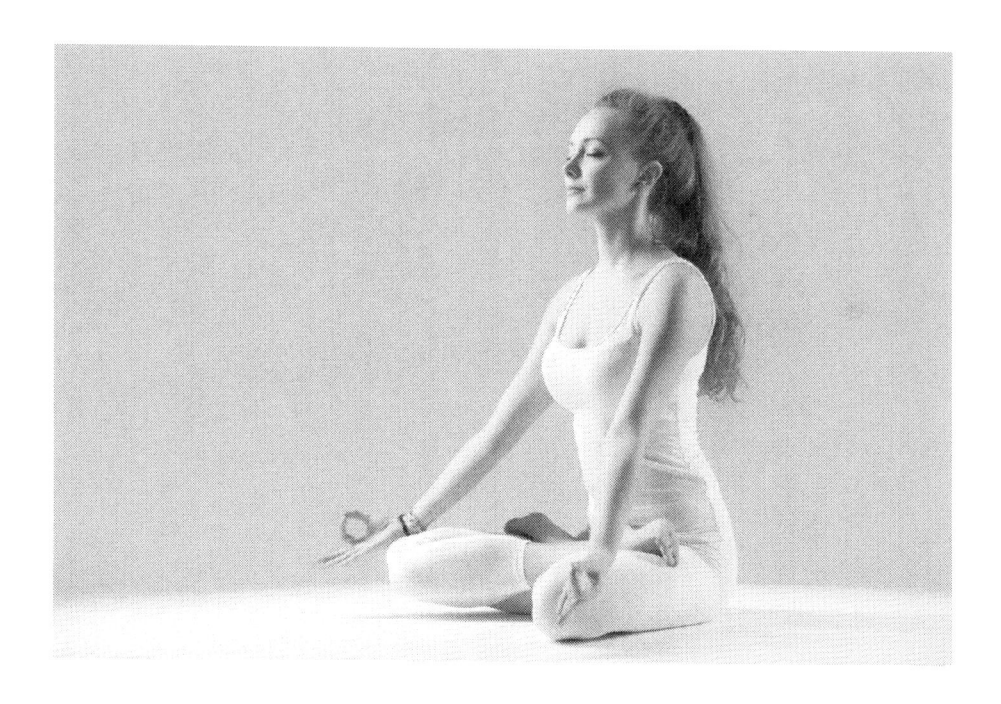

Instructions
1. Sit on the yoga mat with your legs stretched straight.
2. Keep your spine erect.
3. Bend your right leg and place your right foot on the left thigh, close to your hips. Your right heel should be close to your abdomen.
4. Repeat the above step with your left leg. Now your feet are placed on opposite thighs.
5. Rest your hands on your knees, assuming chin mudra. In chin mudra, bring the tips of your index finger and thumb together in slight contact. The remaining three fingers remain outstretched.
6. Keep your eyes closed.
7. Remain in the pose for one minute, initially. Once you get comfortable holding the pose you can increase the duration and remain in the pose for up to 30 minutes or one hour. Lotus pose is ideal for meditation once you can hold the pose comfortably.

Benefits
- Calms the nervous system
- Opens up and strengthens the hips
- Stretches the spine, knees, and ankles
- Tones the back muscles
- Corrects posture
- Relieves menstrual discomfort
- Stimulates the abdominal organs and pelvic area
- Reduces sciatic conditions
- Promotes flexibility of the knees
- Calms the mind
- Improves focus

Caution
Those with chronic injuries in the knees or ankles should refrain from practicing lotus pose. If placing both feet on the opposite thighs is difficult, you may practice with your right foot on top of the left thigh and keep the left leg under the right. This pose is called easy pose (p141).

Thunderbolt Pose

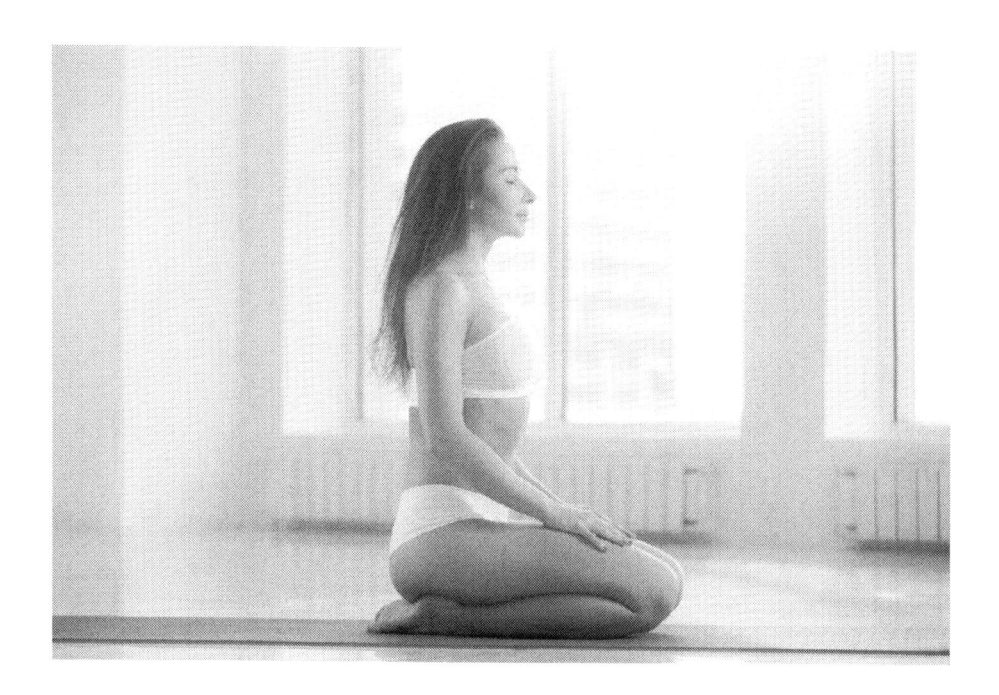

Thunderbolt pose is an exception to the rule that yoga poses should be performed on an empty stomach. This pose can be performed even immediately after eating.

Instructions

1. Kneel down on the mat, with the thighs together.
2. With the big toes touching, spread your heels apart so that your feet form a 'V' shape.
3. Exhale, and place your butt on the space between your feet. Keep the spine straight.
4. Place your palms on your knees.
5. Remain in the pose for one minute.

Benefits

- Improves digestion
- Relieves gas
- Stretches the whole leg

- Massages the pelvic area
- Improves posture
- Promotes calm

Caution

Those with knee or ankle injuries should avoid practicing this pose.

Extended Puppy Pose

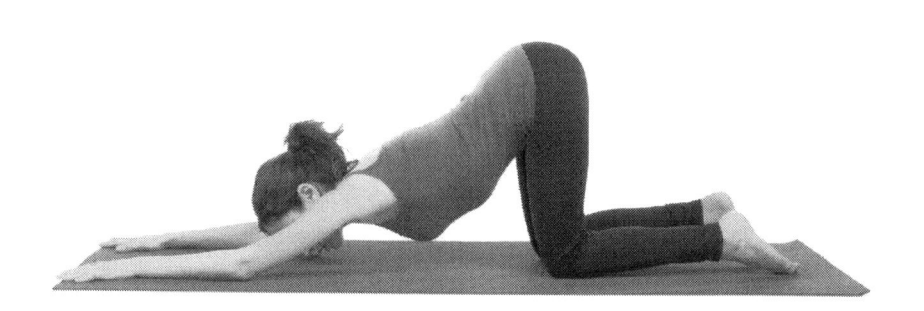

Instructions
1. Come down on all fours. Your wrists should be in line with your shoulders, and your knees with your hips.
2. Walk your hands forward, and lower your chest towards the ground.
3. With your hips over your knees, lengthen your spine and release your forehead to the floor.
4. Expand the shoulders.
5. Inhale, and lift your hips further up towards the ceiling as your chest goes further down, arching your back slightly.
6. Remain in the pose for one minute.
7. To come out of the pose, walk your hands back to the initial position.

Benefits
- Stretches the spine and upper back
- Stretches the shoulders and arms
- Cures insomnia
- Relieves stress and anxiety
- Promotes calm

Note
If placing the forehead on the ground is difficult, place a folded blanket underneath, as the elevation will help you.

Caution
Those with knee injuries should refrain from practicing this pose.

Seated Forward Bend

Seated forward bend is one of the best beginner yoga poses. Though a beginner pose, it may be a little difficult for some. However, with practice the pose can be mastered.

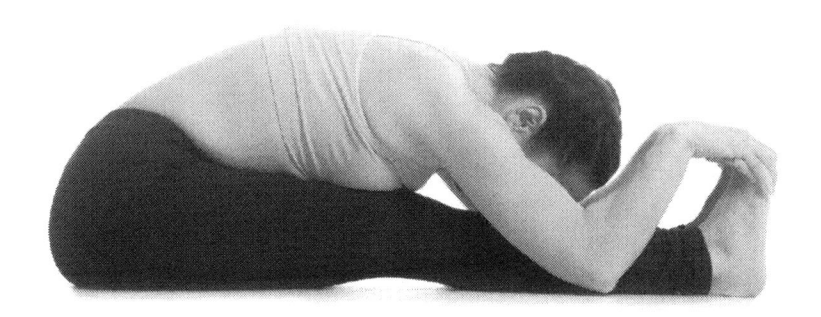

Instructions

1. Sit down with your legs stretched forward. The feet should be straight.
2. Keep your spine erect.
3. Inhale and lift your hands sideways and over your head.
4. Exhale as you bend forward towards your toes.
5. Hold your feet, keeping your legs firmly on the floor.
6. Place your head on your knees, or below. Try to bring your elbows to the floor.
7. Remain in the pose for 30 seconds.
8. Breathe in as you rise up out of the pose.

Benefits
- Stretches the entire back and contracts the inner side
- Stretches and tones the spine
- Tones the back muscles
- Stimulates the function of abdominal organs such as the kidneys, liver, and spleen
- Improves digestion
- Relieves menstrual discomfort
- Regulates blood sugar levels
- Activates Kundalini power
- Calms the brain
- Encourages acceptance

Note

Do not force your body into the pose. If you are unable to reach your feet at first, you can hold your knees or calves. Alternately, you can use a yoga strap. Bend only to the point of slight discomfort. With practice, you will be able to perform the pose to perfection.

Caution

Those with slipped disc conditions or sciatic problems should refrain from practicing this pose.

Bridge Pose

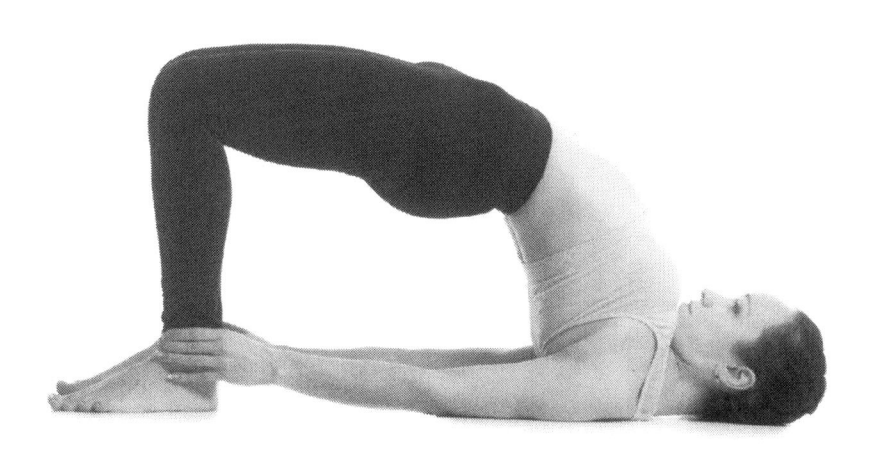

Instructions
1. Lie on your back.
2. Bend your knees and place your feet flat on the floor. Your feet should be in line with your knees, and hip-width apart.
3. Keep your hands by your sides, the palms on the floor.
4. Inhale, and lift your hips off the floor. Your head, neck, shoulders, hands, and feet will be on the floor.
5. Keep your legs and feet parallel to each other.
6. Bring your hands under your back on the floor, and clasp them.
7. Remain in the pose for one minute.
8. To come out of the pose, unclasp your hands, lower your hips to the floor, and stretch your legs.

Benefits
- Opens the chest and shoulders
- Stretches the spine
- Tones the back muscles
- Stretches the hips and thighs
- Improves digestion
- Strengthens respiratory function
- Supports healthy function of the thyroid
- Lowers high blood pressure
- Relieves symptoms of menopause
- Relieves fatigue
- Relieves stress
- Calms the mind

Note
Those with difficulty in holding the hips high, place a block under the back of your pelvis.

Caution
Those with any injury in the shoulders or neck should refrain from practicing this pose.

Upside-Down Seal Yoga Pose

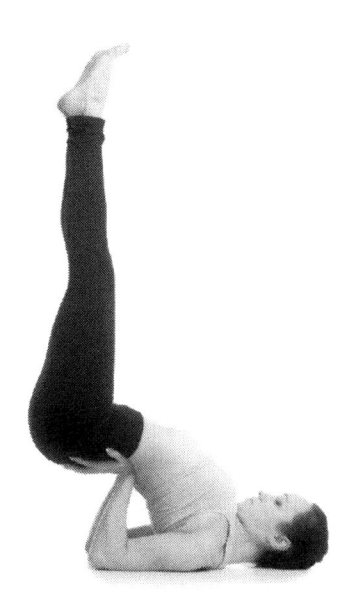

Instructions

1. Lie down on your back with your legs stretched forward. Place your hands by your sides. Inhale.
2. Exhale as you lift your legs at an angle of 90 degrees. Your legs should be perpendicular to your hips. The soles of the feet should face upward.
3. Supporting the hips with your palms, lift the hips further up until the hips are at a 45 degree angle from your shoulders.
4. Look at your toes, or keep the eyes closed.
5. Remain in the pose for one minute. You can gradually increase the duration to 15 minutes.

Benefits

- Promotes blood flow to the head
- Oxygenates the whole body
- Improves lung capacity and cures respiratory disorders
- Strengthens the function of abdominal organs

- Relieves constipation
- Improves digestion
- Postpones the symptoms of aging
- Cures insomnia
- Improves vision
- Relieves menstrual cramps
- Promotes youthfulness

Note
As the name suggests, the pose can be performed using a wall for support. Lie down a few inches from the wall and place your legs on it for support. You can place a pillow, block, or a folded blanket under your hips to help you hold the pose.

Caution
The pose should not be performed during menstruation. Seek professional advice if you have high blood pressure or severe eye conditions. Those with neck, shoulder, or back injuries should perform the pose only with props.

Fire Log Pose

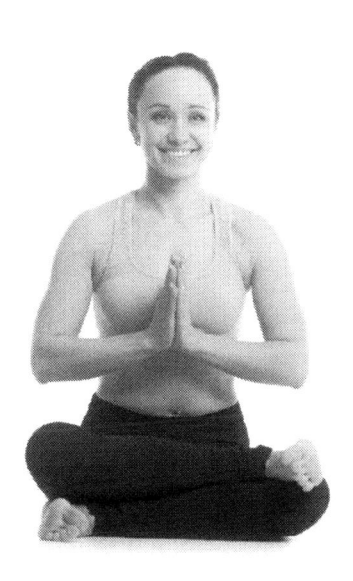

Instructions
1. Sit down with your legs stretched out and your hands by your sides.
2. Bend your left leg and place your foot on the right knee. The right ankle should extend outside the left knee.
3. Slide the right foot under your left knee.
4. Sit straight, lengthening your spine.
5. Place your hands by your sides.
6. Inhale and exhale.
7. Remain in the pose for one minute.
8. Repeat with the right leg on top.

Benefits
- Stretches the hips, thighs, and groin
- Opens the hips
- Stimulates the function of the abdominal organs
- Stretches the calves
- Relieves stress
- Calms the mind

Caution
Those with severe knee or lower back injury should not practice this pose.

Other yoga poses for headache include:
- Big Toe Pose – p105
- Dolphin Pose – p128
- Downward Facing Dog Pose – p88
- Standing Forward Bend – p84

Yoga for Indigestion and Constipation

Indigestion is one of the most common disorders found in the global population. Not only is the condition common, it is also the root cause for various diseases. Yoga helps to cure indigestion by stimulating the digestive organs. It cleanses them, and aids in removing waste. Yoga also relieves stress, a major contributor to the condition. Here are the top beginner yoga poses for indigestion.

Wind Relieving Pose

Wind relieving pose expels gas and stimulates abdominal organs.

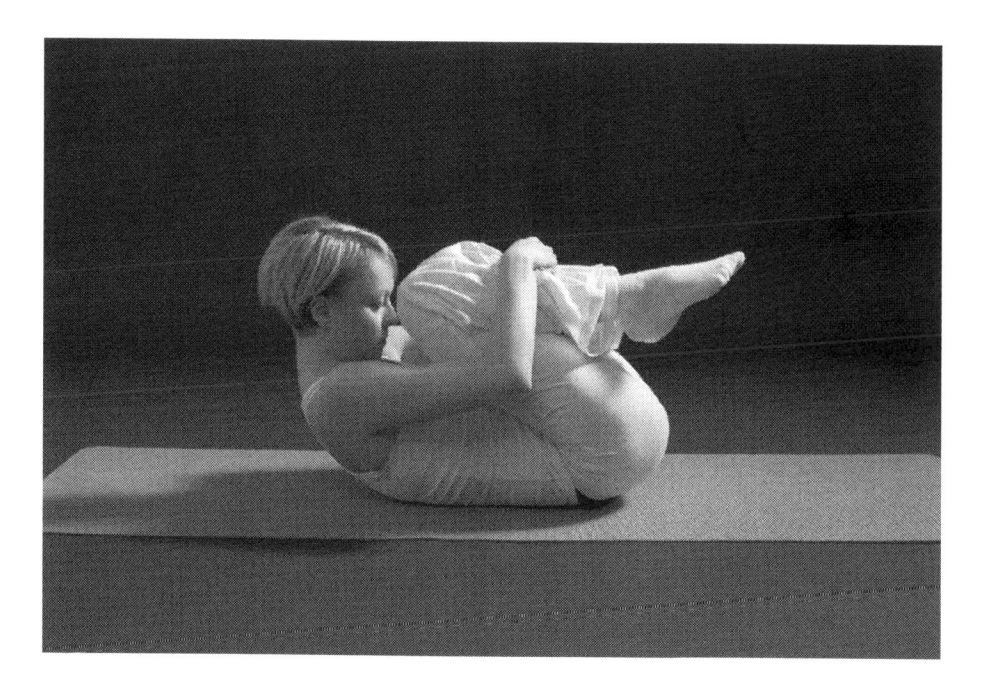

Instructions
1. Lie down on your back with your legs outstretched. Keep your hands by your sides.
2. Inhale as you lift both the legs straight in, drawing the knees toward your face.
3. Place your thighs on your abdomen.
4. Bring your arms over your legs and lock your fingers. You can also hold the elbows of the opposite arms.
5. Pressing your legs into your abdomen, draw the knees closer to your face. Lift your head and bring your chin up to touch your knees. Breathe normally.
6. Remain in the pose for 30 seconds.

Benefits
- Tones the abdominal muscles
- Stretches the spine
- Strengthens the back muscles
- Relieves back pain
- Reduces tummy fat
- Reduces arthritis
- Relieves menstrual disorders
- Stimulates the reproductive organs

Note
If you are unable to touch your chin to your knees, you may place your forehead against your knees instead.

Caution
Those with neck pain should not lift their heads. This pose should not be practiced by those with high blood pressure, heart problems, acidity, hernia, and slipped discs. Those with chronic back and neck problems are also advised against practicing the pose.

Half Tortoise Pose

This is one of the best beginner yoga poses to relieve indigestion and constipation.

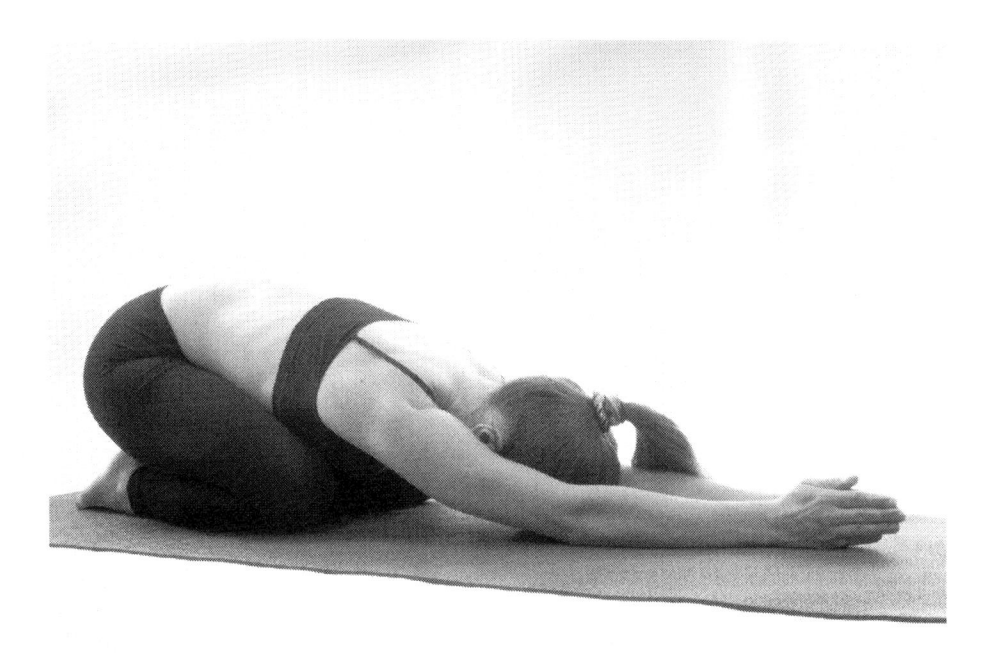

Instructions
1. Sit in thunderbolt pose, in which you will be seated on the space between your heels.
2. With inhalation, lift your arms over your head.
3. Place the palms together and entwine your thumbs. Lengthen the spine and sit straight. Keep your elbows straight so that your biceps touch your ears.
4. With slow exhalation, bend forward at your hips to place your forehead and little fingers on the ground. Breathe normally.
5. Remain in the pose for 30 seconds.
6. To come out of the pose, inhale, lift your body and hands up, and release your arms.

Benefits
- Improves blood circulation to the brain and boosts brain function
- Stretches the spine, shoulders, and hips
- Massages the heart and improves its function
- Improves respiratory function
- Tones the back and the abdominal organs
- Tones the thighs
- Cures insomnia
- Relieves headache
- Regulates blood sugar levels
- Relieves stress

Note
Avoid practicing the pose if you have chronic knee problems.

Head to Knee Pose

Head to Knee Pose tones abdominal organs and supports digestion.

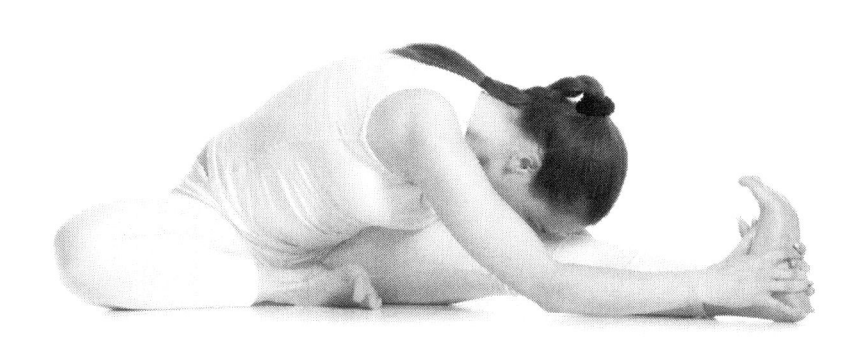

Instructions

1. Sit straight on the mat with your legs stretched forward, with your feet together.
2. Bend your right leg and place your right foot against the inner left thigh on the floor.
3. Your right heel should be close to your perineum.
4. Inhale. Lift your hands to the sides and stretch them over your head with the elbows straight.
5. With exhalation, bend forward with your hands out stretched. Hold the toes of the left leg without bending the knee. Your abdomen should be on the left thigh, and your forehead on or beyond the left knee.
6. Remain in the pose for 30 seconds.
7. Repeat the same steps with the other leg.

Benefits
- Stretches the spine, shoulders, and arms
- Tones the abdominal organs and improves the function of the kidneys and liver
- Relieves sinusitis
- Relieves menstrual disorders and symptoms of PMS
- Relieves headache
- Stimulates the reproductive organs
- Lowers high blood pressure
- Cures insomnia
- Relieves fatigue
- Relieves stress and depression

Note
If you find holding the toes difficult, use a yoga strap around your foot, and hold the ends as you bend forward within your limits.

Caution
Those with heart disease, high blood pressure, chronic back injury, or spondylosis should avoid doing this pose.

Revolved Triangle Pose

Revolved triangle pose is an excellent beginner pose to massage the midsection, relieve constipation, and improve digestion.

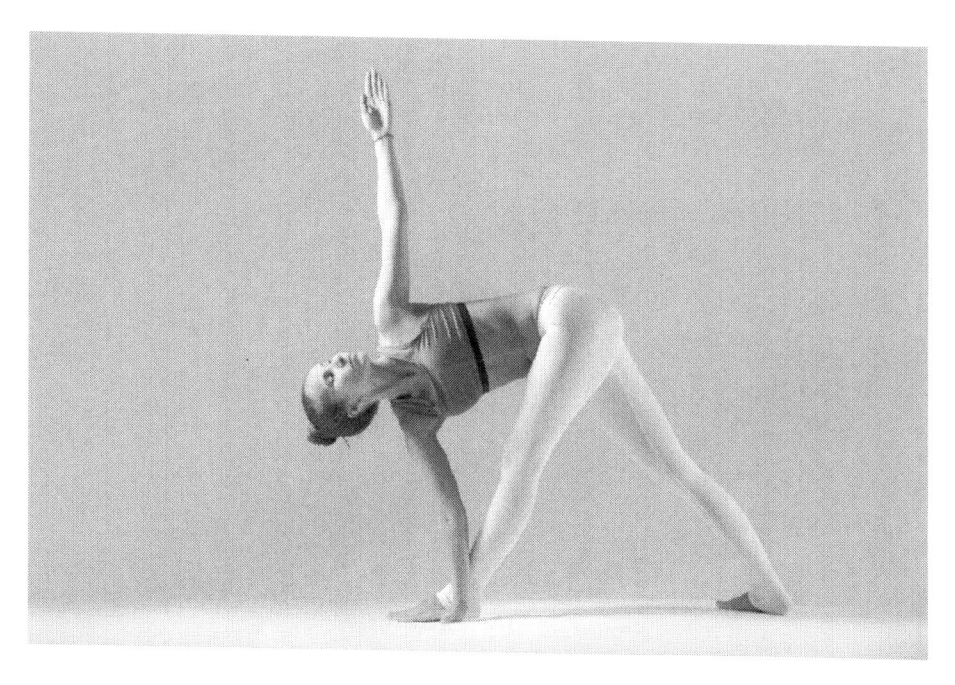

Instructions
1. Stand straight, keeping your hands by your sides.
2. Place your left foot about three to four feet behind your front foot. The left foot should be at 90 degrees and the right foot at about 45 degrees. The heels should be aligned under you.
3. Raise your arms to shoulder level, keeping them parallel to the ground.
4. Exhale as you turn your torso to your right.
5. Square your hips to bring the left hip even with the right.
6. Exhale, and deepen your pose by turning the torso further to the right.
7. Bend forward, towards your right leg. Bring the left hand down and place it on the outer side of the right foot.

8. Stretch your right hand up, with the fingers pointing the ceiling.
9. Turn your face and gaze at the thumb of the extended hand. Beginners can keep their head neutral until balance is achieved.
10. Remain in the pose for one minute.
11. Repeat the steps on the other side.

Benefits
- Opens the chest
- Strengthens respiratory function and relieves respiratory disorders, including asthma
- Stretches the spine and hips
- Stretches and strengthens the legs
- Cures sciatica
- Relieves back pain
- Promotes balance
- Improves your sense of coordination

Note
Beginners can place a block under the arm stretched below.

Caution
This pose is not recommended for those with low blood pressure, headache, diarrhea, back or hip injury, or insomnia.

Half Camel Pose

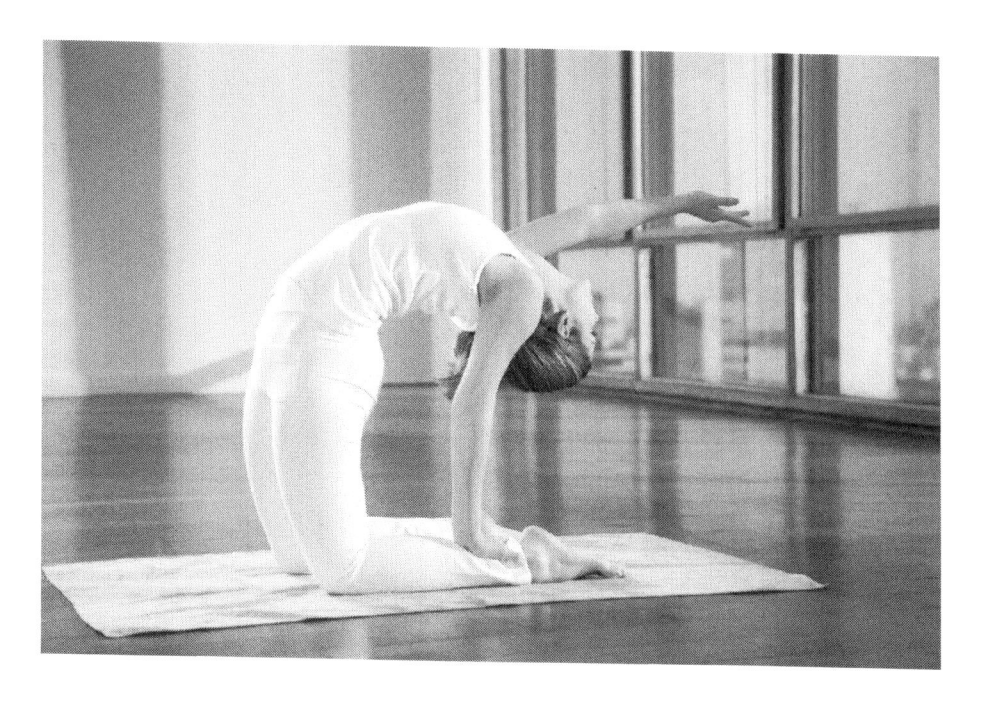

Instructions

1. Go down on your knees. Keep your knees and feet hip-width apart.
2. Place your palms on your hips
3. Inhale as you lengthen the spine and move your hips forward.
4. Lower your right hand and hold the right heel.
5. Inhale and lift your left hand up and backwards so the fingers are pointed towards the wall behind you.
6. Gently drop the head as you arch your back and lift your arm.
7. Remain in the pose for 30 seconds.
8. Come out of the pose by straightening your back and neck and releasing your arms to hold the hips.
9. Repeat the same steps on the other side.

Note
Those who cannot reach their heels can place their hands on their hips.

Caution
Avoid practicing the pose if you have hernia, or a chronic hip or back injury.

Half Plough Pose

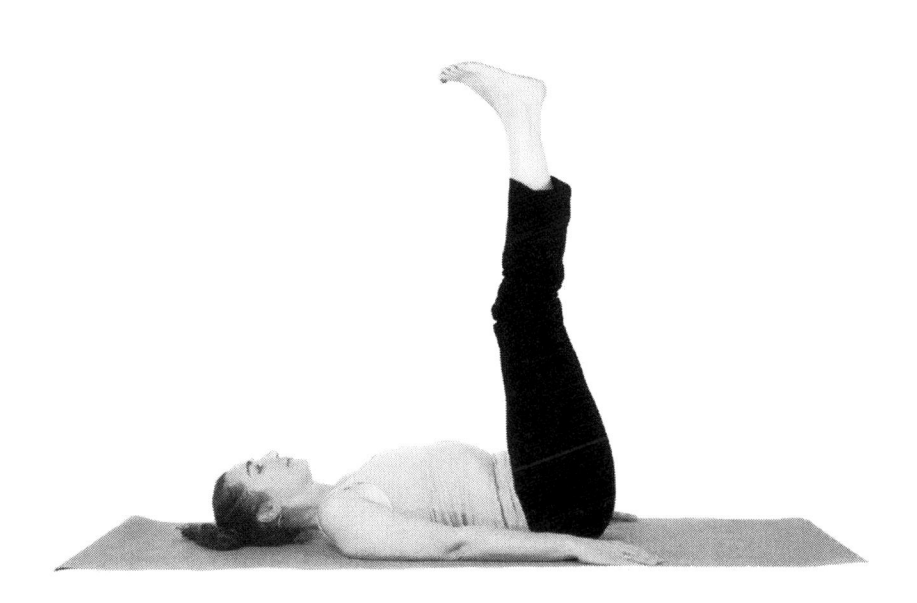

Instructions
1. Lie down on your back, keep legs together, and arms relaxed to the side of the thighs. Place palm facing down.
2. Slowly breathe in and raise both legs up.
3. Keep the knees straight.
4. Hold your breath and stay in this position as long as possible.
5. Breathe out and bring slowly your legs to the floor.
6. Relax for a moment and repeat the pose for 3 to 5 times.

Benefits
- Improves digestion and appetite.
- Improves blood circulation.
- Strengthens the thigh muscles and calf muscles.
- Helps to reduce abdomen fat and to lose weight.
- Stimulates the abdominal organs.

Caution
Avoid practicing if you have a cardiac problem, back pain, or high blood pressure.

Yoga for Asthma

Asthma, a chronic lung disease, is effectively treated by yoga. Yoga poses strengthen the respiratory system and promote the flow of oxygen. Certain yoga poses are excellent chest openers that promote healthy lungs and heart. Breathing techniques in yoga promote slow and deep breathing, which can help calm the sufferer. Yoga poses relieve stress, which can also trigger asthma attack.

Given below are the most effective beginner poses for asthma.

The Psychic Union Pose

Also called forward bend sitting on heels, this pose stimulates the lungs, improves respiratory function, and relieves tightness in the chest.

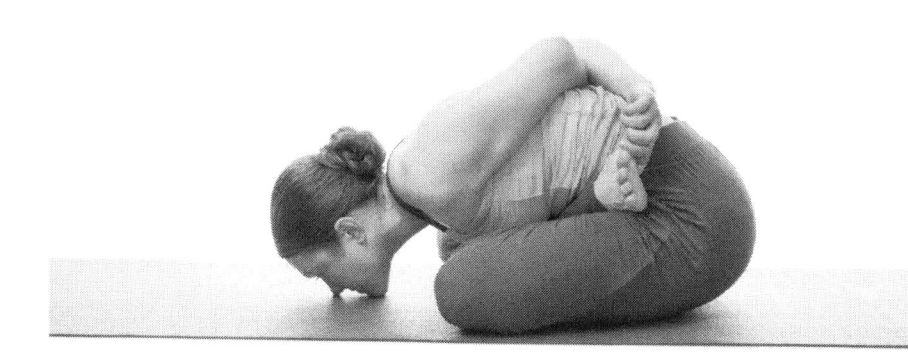

Instructions
1. Sit in lotus pose.
2. Inhale, stretch your arms above you, and bring them behind your back.
3. Hold the left wrist with your right hand. For a more advanced challenge, you may hold the toes of the opposite legs by crossing your hands at the back.
4. Exhale, lengthen your spine, and bend forward to place your forehead on the ground. Do not lift your buttocks.
5. Inhale and exhale.
6. Remain in the pose for 30 seconds to one minute.
7. To come out of the pose, breathe in as you straighten your back.

Benefits
- Improves blood flow to the brain
- Strengthens the abdominal muscles
- Improves digestion
- Relieves constipation
- Improves appetite
- Lengthens the spine
- Tones the back muscles
- Reduces tummy fat
- Promotes hip flexibility
- Reduces thigh fat
- Regulates blood sugar levels
- Increases focus

Caution
Those with a chronic back injury should avoid practicing this pose. Those with heart conditions or severe eye problems should also avoid this pose.

Shoulder Stand

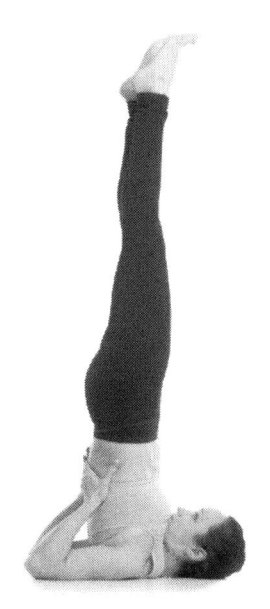

Shoulder stand is referred to as the queen of all asanas. The pose increases lung capacity and promotes lung function, thereby relieving the symptoms of respiratory disorders, including asthma. It also boosts immunity, thereby reducing and preventing attacks of asthma.

Instructions
1. Lie down on your back, stretching your legs straight. Keep your hands by your sides.
2. Exhale, and lift your legs with one swift move so that your buttocks, hips, and back are completely raised.
3. Support your hips by placing your palms behind you. Your elbows should be behind your back and close to each other. Move the palms up closer to the shoulder blades to straighten your stand.
4. Keep the legs straight and your toes pointed upwards.
5. Bring your sternum to your chin.
6. Breathe deeply.

7. Remain in the pose for one minute.
8. To release the pose, bring your knees towards your forehead. Place your arms on the floor, palms down. Release your spine to allow your body to come to the floor. Lower your legs, and stretch them on the floor.

Benefits
- Cures and prevents cold and cough
- Promotes blood circulation
- Supports the function of the glands
- Helps maintain a healthy body weight
- Strengthens the nervous system
- Improves digestion
- Improves immunity
- Strengthens the neck
- Strengthens the reproductive system
- Aids in detoxification
- Promotes calm

Note
Use a folded blanket under your neck if the pose hurts your neck. You may place your legs on a wall if you find straightening your legs difficult.

Caution
The pose should not be performed by those with heart problems, high blood pressure, slipped disc conditions, cervical spondylitis, or enlarged liver or spleen. Those with severe eye problems should also avoid practicing this pose.

Do not perform the pose during menstruation.

Fish Pose

Fish pose improves lung function and aids in reducing the symptoms of respiratory conditions. It also boosts immunity, thereby helping prevent asthma attacks.

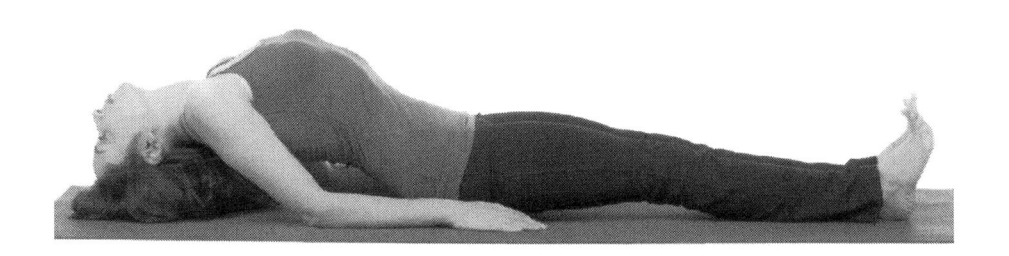

Instructions
1. Lie down on the mat with your legs outstretched and your hands by your sides.
2. Bring your hands behind your head and place the palms on the floor behind your shoulders. The fingers should be pointing to your shoulders.
3. Inhale, and press the palms firmly on the ground, lifting your head and placing the crown on the floor. Arch your back well.
4. Relax the arms to your sides, or tuck the hands under your buttocks.
5. Remain in the pose for about 3 minutes.
6. To release the pose, place your hands behind your shoulders and pressing the palms firmly, lift your hips and release the head and back.

Benefits
- Stretches the chest and improves lung capacity
- Stretches and strengthens the neck and back
- Reduces back pain
- Relieves constipation
- Cures menstrual pain
- Stimulates the function of the glands
- Improves posture

Note
Beginners can use a pillow to support the arch of the back. With practice, the pose can be performed with the legs in lotus position.

Caution
The pose is not recommended for those with insomnia, high or low blood pressure, or severe injury to the neck or back. Avoid this pose if you have a headache.

Other poses that aid in curing asthma include:
- Easy Pose – p141
- Bridge Pose – p168
- Cobra Pose – p71

Yoga for Neck Pain

A good percentage of the world's population suffer from neck pain. The muscles of the neck seem to be the prime target of stress, which can cause severe pain and compromised neck mobility. Owing to current lifestyles, which often involve being seated most of the time, we often have incorrect posture, which also causes neck pain. Yoga stretches, lengthens, relaxes, and strengthens the neck muscles, thereby relieving neck pain.

Some top yoga poses for neck pain are shown below.

Easy Pose with Twist

Easy Pose with Twist, as the name suggests, is a variation of Easy Pose. It stretches and strengthens the neck muscles thereby relieving neck pain.

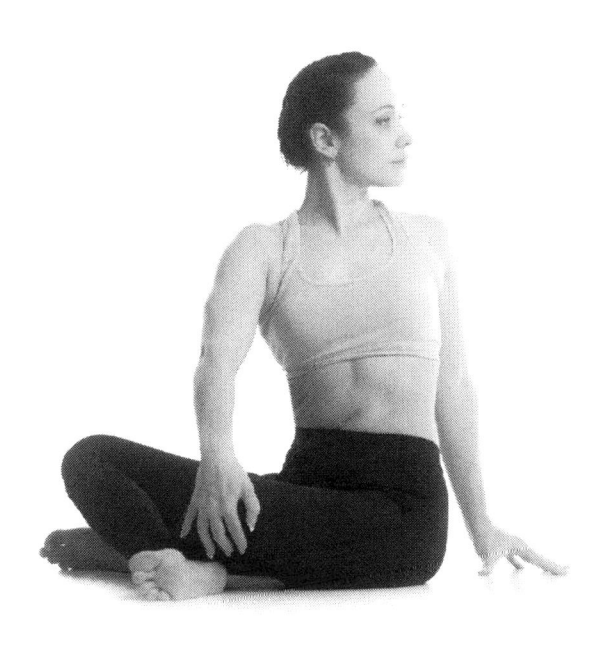

Instructions
1. Assume easy pose, in which you sit straight with the legs crossed at the shins.
2. Keep your body weight balanced evenly on the sit bones.
3. Lengthen your spine and keep the neck relaxed.
4. Lift your right hand and bring it behind your back, to place the palm on the floor behind your right buttock. Maintain a few inches of space between your palm and butt.
5. With exhalation, gently twist your torso to your right as you place the left hand on the outer side of your right knee.
6. Turn your head to your right and gaze over your right shoulder. Keep your shoulders open.
7. With every inhalation and exhalation, deepen the pose by twisting. Only twist to the extent your flexibility allows.
8. Remain in the pose for one minute.
9. Repeat the same steps on the other side.

Benefits
- Stretches the shoulders, back, hips, and knees
- Increases spine flexibility
- Relieves shoulder pain
- Energizes the whole body
- Improves digestion
- Tones the back muscles and abdominal organs
- Relieves stress

Note
Those with tight hips can elevate the hips by placing a pillow or a block under the hips. This will help you twist your torso more easily.

Caution
Avoid practicing the pose if you have severe knee or hip conditions.

Seated Eagle Pose

Seated eagle pose is a variation and simpler version of eagle pose. Seated eagle pose relieves stress in the neck.

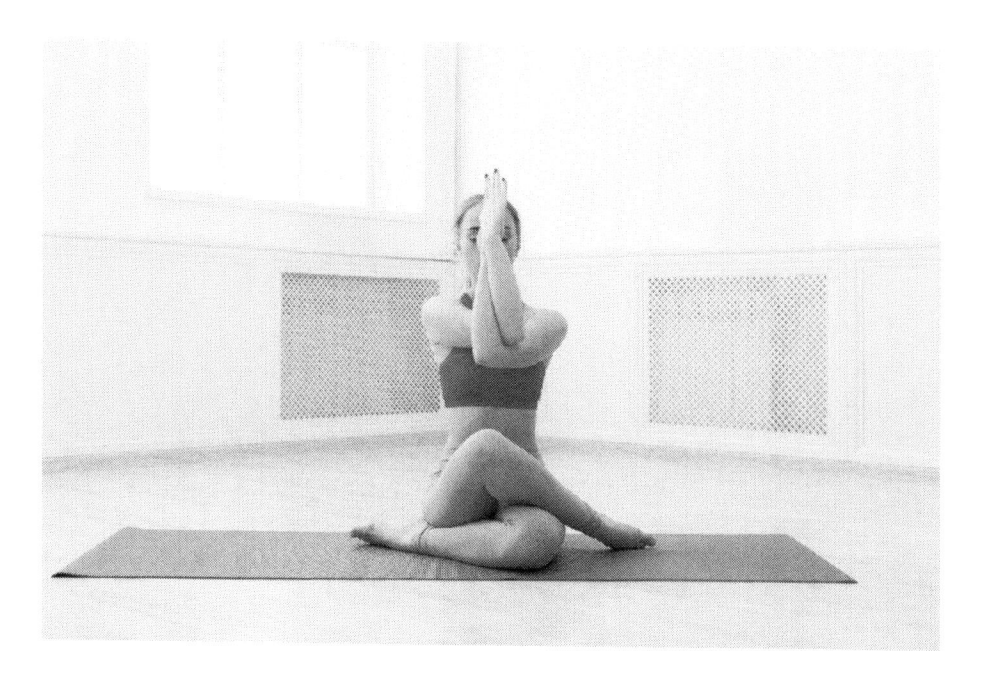

Instructions
1. Sit on the floor in lotus pose or easy pose, whichever is more comfortable for you.
2. Bring your arms in front of you, keeping the hands close together.
3. Wrap your right arm around your left arm by placing the right over the left and curling it. Place the palms against each other. The intertwined arms will resemble two snakes.
4. Keep your shoulders relaxed.
5. Look straight ahead.
6. Remain in the pose for about 3 minutes.
7. Come out of the pose by releasing the arms and placing your hands on your thighs.
8. Repeat the same process with the left hand wrapping the right.

Benefits
- Stretches the shoulders and arms
- Opens up the shoulders
- Corrects the posture of the upper back
- Relieves stress in the shoulders
- Straightens the spine
- Promotes balance
- Boosts willpower

Caution
Those with chronic shoulder or elbow injury should refrain from practicing this pose.

Twisted Pose

Also called simple spinal twist, twisted pose is another beginner poses that is effective in relieving neck pain. It stretches and tones the neck.

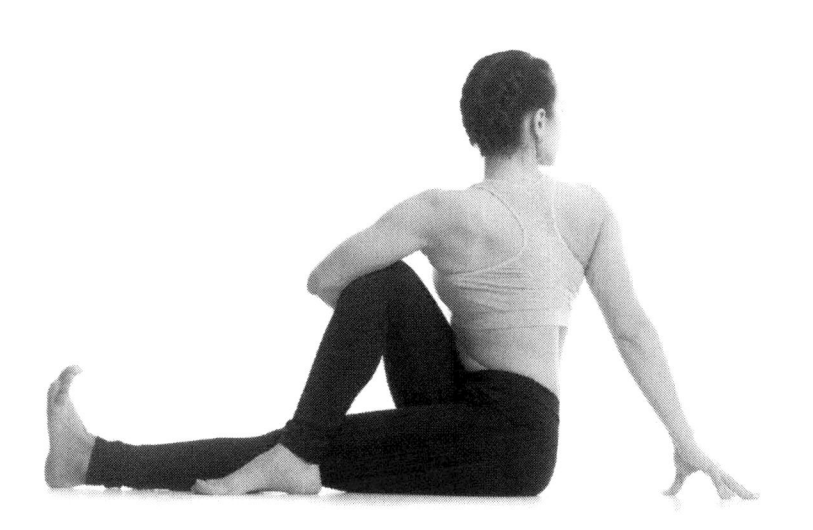

Instructions
1. Sit down with the legs stretched forward.
2. Exhale. Bend your right leg and place your right foot by the outer side of your left knee.
3. With inhalation, place your right hand behind your right buttock, with your fingers pointing outwards.
4. Exhale as you twist your torso to your right.
5. Bring your left hand over your right knee towards your right side.
6. Try to align your shoulder blades with your extended leg.
7. Remain in the pose for 30 seconds.
8. Repeat the same with the other leg.

Benefits
- Increases spine flexibility
- Tones the back muscles
- Stimulates the abdominal organs
- Improves digestion
- Relieves constipation
- Reduces tummy fat
- Relaxes the hips and knees
- Stimulates the solar plexus chakra

Caution
Those with any spine injury, ulcer, or hip and knee injuries should avoid practicing this pose.

Other poses for relieving neck pain include:
- Extended Triangle Pose - p133 (Instructions in 'Core' category)
- Child's Pose –p145 (Instructions in 'Headache' category)
- Fish Pose – p189

Yoga for Back Pain

Back pain may be caused by various factors, including injury, muscle strain, bad posture, lifting heavy weights awkwardly, or lifting even a near-weightless object in an awkward bend – and sitting day in and day out. Yoga helps to relieve back pain, as the poses tone the back muscles, strengthen the spine, and improve flexibility. Practicing yoga also helps to prevent injuries. Yoga makes you aware of your body, your posture, and corrects your posture to save your back.

Here are the most effective beginner yoga poses for back pain.

Sphinx Pose

Sphinx Pose is a basic backbend pose that is highly effective for back pain. It reverses the ill effects caused to the lower back due to prolonged sitting.

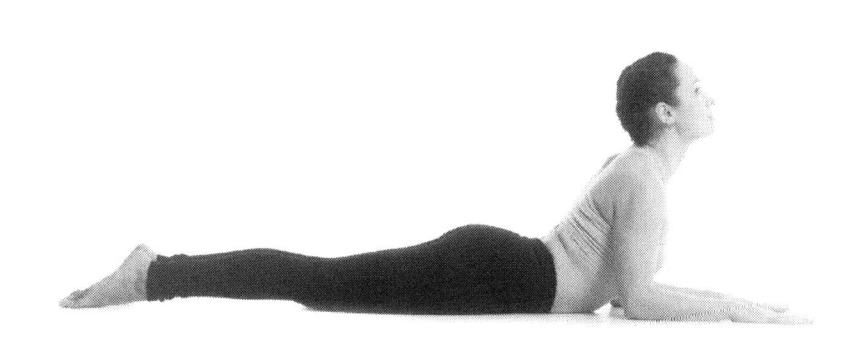

Instructions
1. Lie down on your stomach.
2. Maintain a hip-width distance between your feet.
3. Draw your hands forward to place the forearms on the floor, aligning the elbows with the shoulders. Arch your upper body gently upward.
4. Remain in the pose for 3 minutes.
5. To release the pose, place your upper body on the floor and straighten your arms.

Benefits
- Strengthens the spine
- Stretches the front of the upper body
- Stimulates lung function
- Tones the abdominal organs
- Improves digestion
- Energizes the body
- Calms the nervous system
- Relieves fatigue

Note
If you find holding the pose difficult, you may move your arms a bit forward from your shoulders to reduce the impact the pose has on your back. On the contrary, if your flexibility allows you to go deeper into the pose, place blocks under the elbows.

Caution
Avoid practicing the pose if you have severe injury to your back, shoulders, or arms.

Rabbit Pose

Counter to sphinx pose, rabbit pose requires bending your back forward. It is an excellent beginner pose to stretch and strengthen your back muscles.

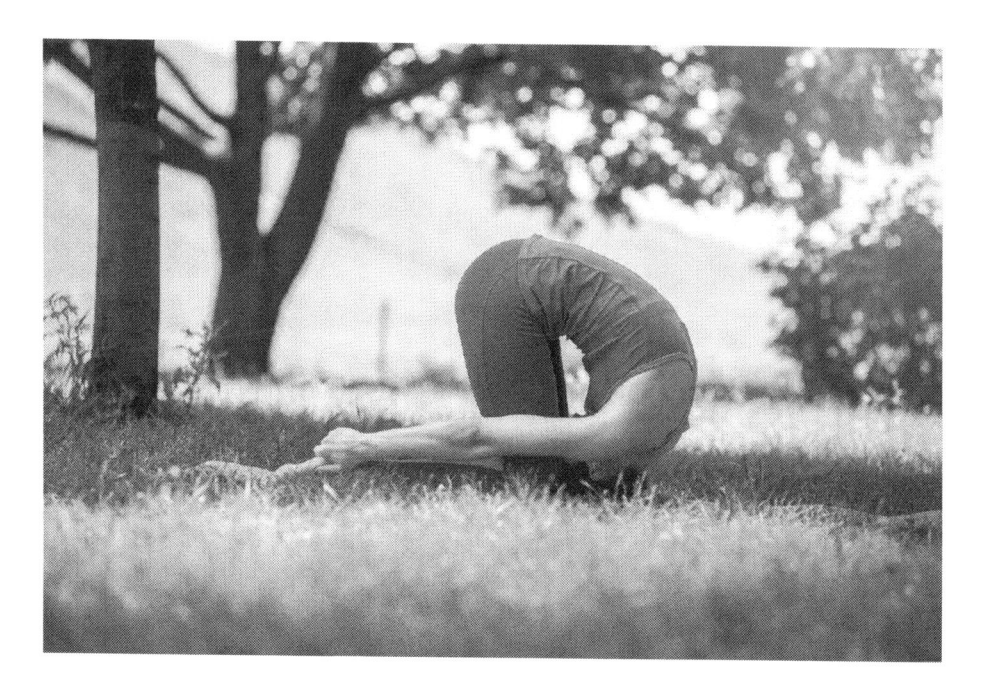

Instructions
1. Sit on your heels. Keep the knees hip-width apart.
2. Inhale and bring your hands back to hold your heels. The heels should be held in such a way that the back of the hand should be facing the outer sides, and the fingers should be on the heels with the thumb close to the fingers, but at the side.
3. With exhalation, tuck your chin in and gently bend forward.
4. Place the crown of your head on the floor in front of your knees.
5. Breathing normally, lift your buttocks high to keep your thighs almost vertical to the floor.

6. Keep your chin locked to your chest.
7. Remain in the pose for one minute.
8. Come out of the pose by lowering your back and then releasing your heels.

Benefits
- Releases stress in the neck and shoulders
- Stretches the spine, shoulders, and arms
- Stimulates the thyroid and parathyroid glands
- Helps maintains a healthy metabolism
- Boosts immune function
- Tones the abdominal organs
- Improves digestion
- Corrects posture
- Cures insomnia
- Relieves depression

Note
Do not apply pressure on your crown and neck. You may place a folded blanket under your knees to prevent your knees from hurting.

Caution
Those with chronic conditions in the neck, shoulder, spine, or knees should refrain from practicing this pose.

Upward Plank Pose

Upward plank pose is a mild backbend pose that supports the spine and protects back health.

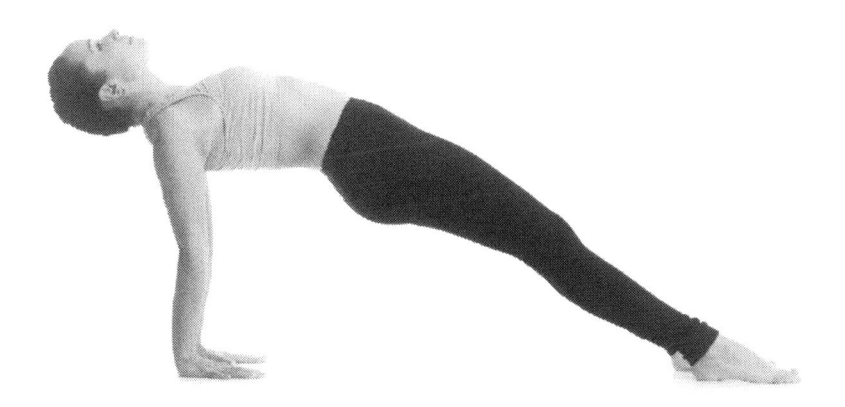

Instructions
1. Sit straight with your legs extended in front of you.
2. Place your hands behind your hips on the floor, a few inches away from your buttocks. Your fingers should be pointed forward.
3. With your hands and feet firmly on the ground, lift your sternum off the floor as high as possible, so your body curves into a mild backbend.
4. Tuck in your chin to your chest.
5. Gently drop your head back, giving your neck a nice stretch.
6. Remain in the pose for 30 seconds.
7. To come out of the pose, bring your head straight and release your hips to the floor.

Benefits
- Stretches and strengthens the arms and wrists
- Stretches and strengthens the shoulders, chest, and legs
- Stretches the spine
- Calms the mind

Caution
Avoid practicing the pose if you have injuries in the neck or wrists.

Other poses that relieve back pain include:
- Cat Pose – p111
- Cow Pose – p109
- Camel Pose – p115
- Tree Pose – p86
- Bow Pose – p113

Yoga for Menstrual Disorders and Menopause

Yoga is great for women, as it addresses menstrual disorders and relieves the symptoms of menopause. Yoga promotes blood flow and oxygen flow. It stimulates organs and glands, and boosts their performance. It aids in maintaining hormonal balance, thereby alleviating PMS, mood swings, and depression, which are also caused by an imbalance of hormones. Yoga cures headache, menstrual cramps, abdominal pain, and backache. Yoga calms your mind and relieves stress and mood swings.

Half Moon Pose

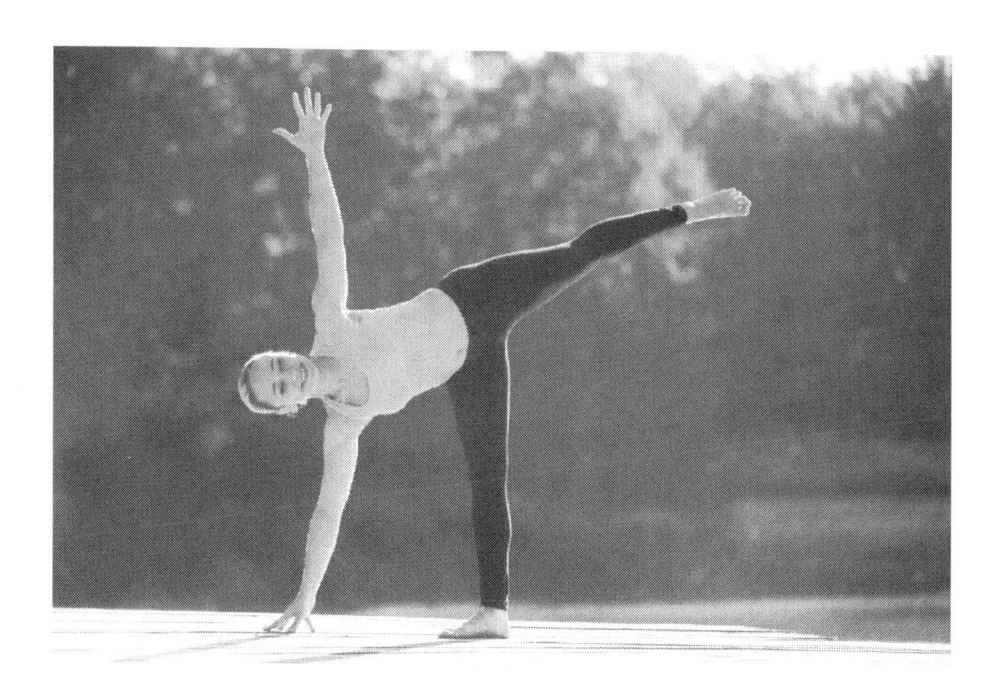

Instructions
1. Stand with your feet wide apart.
2. Stretch your arms out to your sides at shoulder level.
3. Turn your right foot 90 degrees outwards from your body, and your left foot slightly towards your right. The right heel should be in line with your left arch.
4. Bending at the right hip, place your right hand on the outer side of the right ankle.
5. Your shoulders should be in one line, that is, the left shoulder should be directly above the right.
6. Place your left hand on your hip.
7. With the right hand firmly placed on the ground, straighten your right leg while lifting the left leg off the floor. Your left leg should be parallel to floor and your left hip should be directly over the right hip.
8. Lift your left hand so your fingers point upwards.
9. Turn your head to look at the thumb of the left hand.
10. Remain in the pose for one minute.
11. Repeat the same with the other hand and leg.

Benefits
1. Relieves menstrual pain
2. Cures back pain
3. Stretches and strengthens the legs and spine
4. Stretches and strengthens the abdominal muscles
5. Lengthens the spine
6. Tones the back and relieves back pain
7. Relieves constipation
8. Improves digestion
9. Increases fertility
10. Relieves fatigue

Note
Since the pose can be slightly challenging for beginners, you can place a block under the arm that is extended towards the floor. You can also practice the pose close to a wall, to support your leg that is parallel to floor. Those with neck pain should look ahead instead of turning the head.

Caution
Those with insomnia or low blood pressure should avoid practicing the pose. Do not practice the pose when you are experiencing headache or diarrhea.

Extended Side Angle Pose

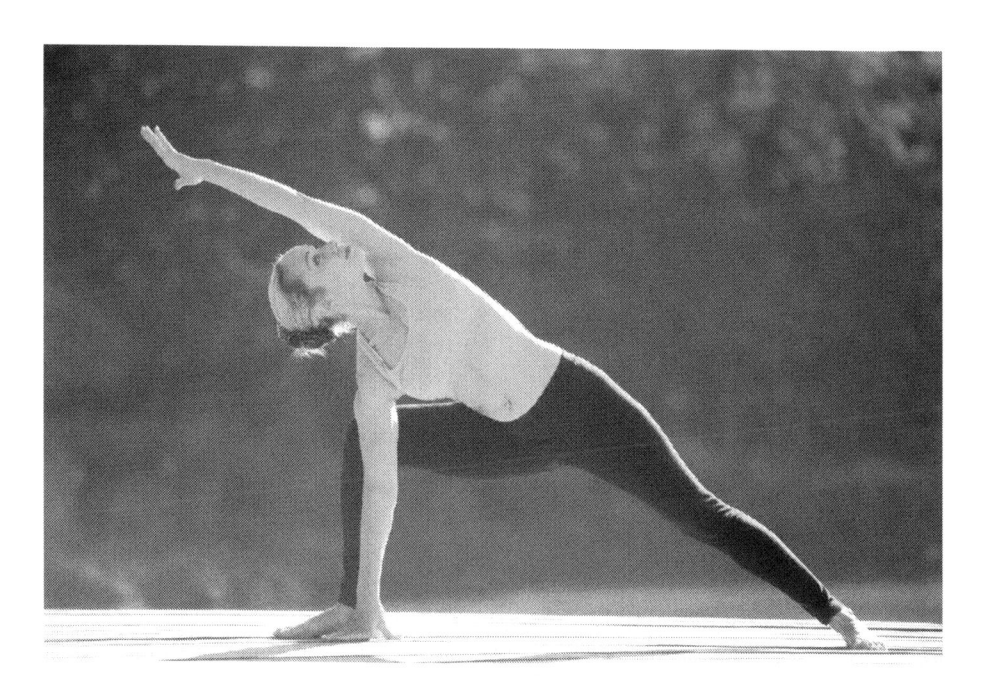

Instructions
1. Stand straight. Keep your feet four to five feet apart, depending on your height and flexibility.
2. Stretch your arms out sideways at shoulder level with the palms facing down. Your wrists should align with your ankles.
3. Turn your right leg 90 degrees to your right. Turn your left toes slightly towards your right.
4. Bend your right knee, keeping your calf perpendicular to the floor. The left leg should be kept straight.
5. Exhale as you bring your right arm to the floor and place the palm close to the side of your right toe. Your forearm should be aligned with your lower leg.
6. Lift your left arm upwards so the fingers point to the ceiling.

7. Go deeper into the stretch, and extend your left arm to your right and beyond your head so the left bicep is over your left ear. The fingers of the left hand should be pointed in the direction your right toes are pointing.
8. Do not bend forward. Your chest, hips, and the stretched leg should be in one straight line.
9. Turn your head to look upwards.
10. Remain in the pose for one minute.
11. To come out of the pose, press your back foot firmly to the ground and rise to a standing position. Lower your arms to your sides.
12. Repeat the same steps with the other leg and hand.

Benefits
- Relieves lower back pain and menstrual discomfort
- Relaxes the shoulders and back
- Stretches the spine, chest, abdomen, hips, and legs
- Strengthens the entire body
- Relieves constipation
- Relieves sciatica and osteoporosis
- Boosts stamina

Note
If you have trouble reaching the floor, place your elbow on the thigh of the leg that is bent. You can also place a pillow or block under your hand to increase the height for easy reach.

Caution
Those with low or high blood pressure or insomnia should refrain from practicing this pose. Do not do this pose if you have a headache. Those with any injury to the neck, shoulders, hips, or knees should not practice this pose.

Reclining Hero Pose

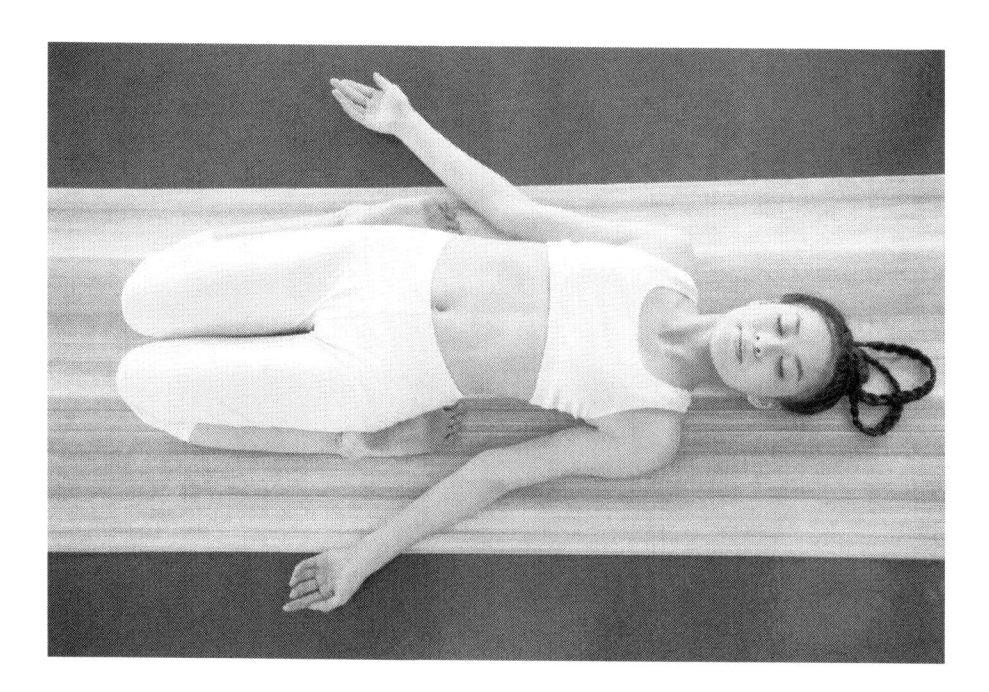

Instructions

1. Assume hero pose, in which you go on your knees, lower your torso, and sit on the space between your heels, keeping the thighs together.
2. Bring your hands behind you, and place them on the floor.
3. Lean back, placing your forearms on the floor.
4. Lean back more, placing the back and the head on the floor. Keep your thighs together without lifting them off the floor.
5. Place your arms by your sides. Alternately, you can bring them over your head on the floor and bend them, holding the elbows with the opposite hands.
6. Remain in the pose for one minute.
7. While coming out of the pose, hold your ankles, and use your forearms to support you while you sit up, again on the space between your heels.

Benefits
- Relieves menstrual cramps and leg pain
- Stretches the back, abdomen, and pelvic region
- Cures asthma
- Improves digestion
- Lowers high blood pressure
- Relieves acidity and gas
- Relieves diarrhea
- Relieves sciatica and varicose veins
- Helps with flat feet

Note
If lying on your back is difficult for you initially, you may rest on the forearms. You can also place a pillow behind your back and rest your back on it.

Caution
Those with heart problems should not practice this pose. Avoid performing the pose if you have a headache. Those with any injury to the back, knees, or ankles should perform the pose only under guidance, and only within the confines of their own comfort.

Reclining Hand-To-Big-Toe Pose

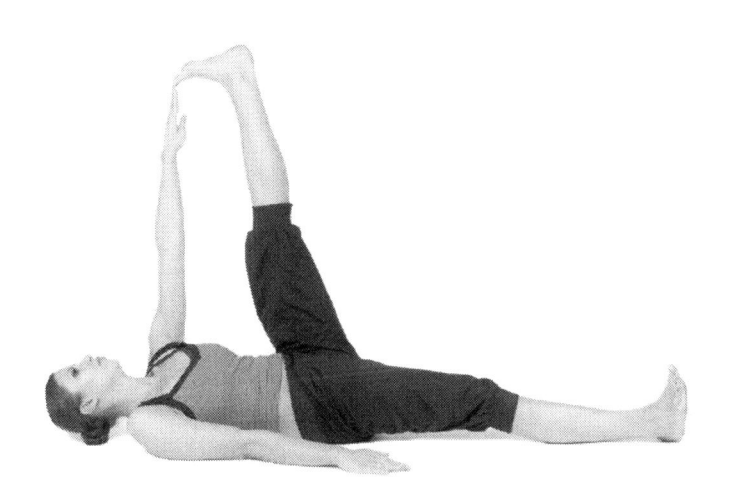

Instructions

1. Lie down on the floor with your legs stretched out and your arms by your sides.
2. Exhale. Bend your right leg and draw the thigh over your torso, hugging the thigh closer to your abdomen.
3. Hold the big toe of your right foot with your thumb, index finger, and middle finger.
4. Gently straighten your right leg and lift it high up towards the ceiling. Maintain a good stretch between your crown and your tailbone.
5. Remain in the pose for 30 seconds.
6. Come out of the pose by placing the lifted leg back down on the floor.
7. Repeat the same steps with the other leg.

Benefits
- Cures back pain, leg pain, and cramps caused by the menstrual cycle
- Stretches the hips, thighs, calves, and hamstrings
- Improves digestion
- Strengthens the knees
- Improves fertility
- Helps with flat feet

Note
You can use a yoga strap to hold your feet if you have difficulty reaching your big toe.
Those with high blood pressure can place a folded blanket under the head.

Caution
Do not practice the pose if you have a hamstring tear. Those with knee pain should not push themselves to hold the toe. Avoid practicing the pose if you are experiencing headache or diarrhea.

Yoga for Relieving Gas

While relieving gas is a normal process, if it exceeds 14 times a day, it should be checked by a doctor. The cause of excess gas could be anything from indigestion to certain medical conditions. Luckily, yoga treats the issue effectively. Certain yoga poses stimulate peristalsis, thereby aiding in releasing excess gas. Yoga boosts blood flow to your digestive system, which aids in healthy digestion and helps prevent the formation of gas. Twists in yoga help cure bloating. Regular practice of yoga keeps your digestive system healthy.

Supine Spinal Twist

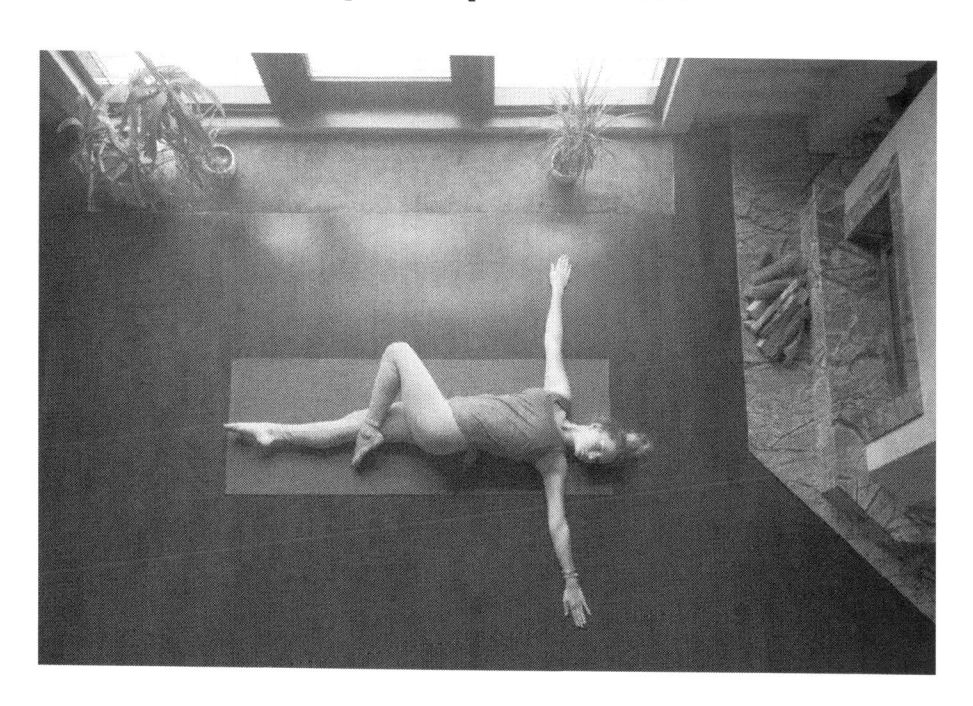

Instructions
1. Lie down on your back. Keep your legs straight and your arms by your sides.
2. Bend your right leg and place the right foot on the left knee.
3. Exhale, and twist your spine to your left, sliding the right knee further to the left side.
4. Your left leg will be nearly straight.
5. Keep the arms aligned with your shoulders.
6. Stretch your right hand straight and the place the left hand on the right knee. You can also keep your arms stretched out at shoulder level.
7. Turn your head towards your right. Fix your gaze on the fingertips of your right hand.
8. Remain in the pose for 30 seconds.
9. Repeat the same steps on the other side.

Benefits
- Stretches and tones the spine
- Stretches the back muscles
- Promotes blood flow to digestive organs
- Relieves gas
- Aids in detoxification

Caution
Those with injury to back, hips and knees should avoid practicing the pose.

Wide-Legged Forward Bend Pose

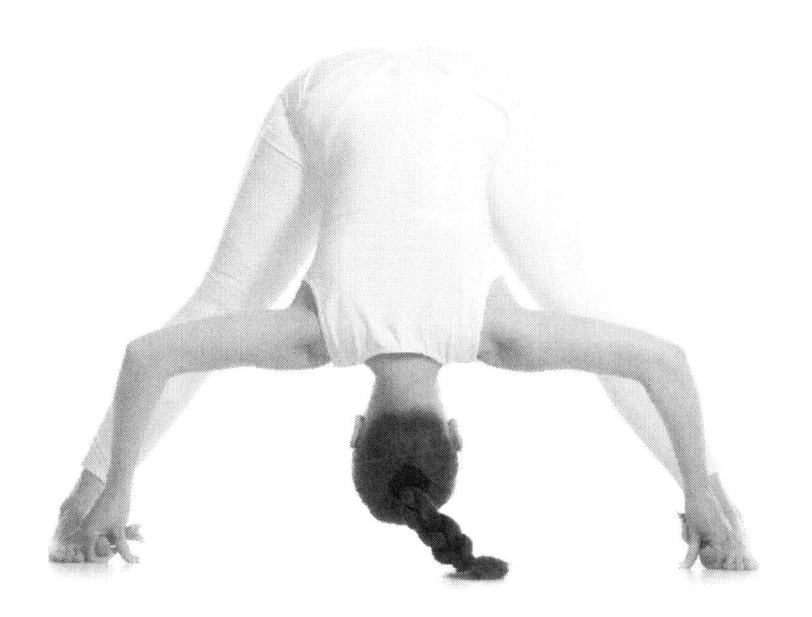

Instructions
1. Stand straight, with your legs four feet apart.
2. Bring your toes slightly in, so your feet are parallel to the sides of the mat. Keep your heels aligned.
3. Inhale, and stretch the upper part of your body upwards.
4. Exhale as you fold forward at the hips.
5. Gently drop your head, and fix your gaze behind you.
6. Place your hands on the floor, shoulder-width apart. If you like, you can grip the big toes of your feet.
7. Go deeper into the pose with an exhale, stretching your torso further down so that your head gets closer to the floor. Those with higher flexibility levels can place the crown of the head on the floor.
8. Bend your elbows. Your elbows should be aligned vertically with your wrists.
9. Remain in the pose for one minute.
10. Release the pose by pressing the feet firmly onto the mat, and straightening your upper body with an inhale.

Benefits
- Tones the abdominal organs, improves digestion, relieves gas
- Relieves tension in the neck, shoulders, back, and hips
- Stretches the shoulders and arms
- Stretches the spine
- Tones the back and relieves minor back pain
- Stretches and strengthens the legs
- Opens the hips
- Relieves stress
- Calms the mind

Note
If stretching down is difficult, place blocks under your arms so you won't need to bend so far. Those with tight hamstrings can bend their knees so their hands can reach the floor or blocks comfortably.

Caution
Avoid practicing the pose if you have a back or hip injury.

Lizard Pose

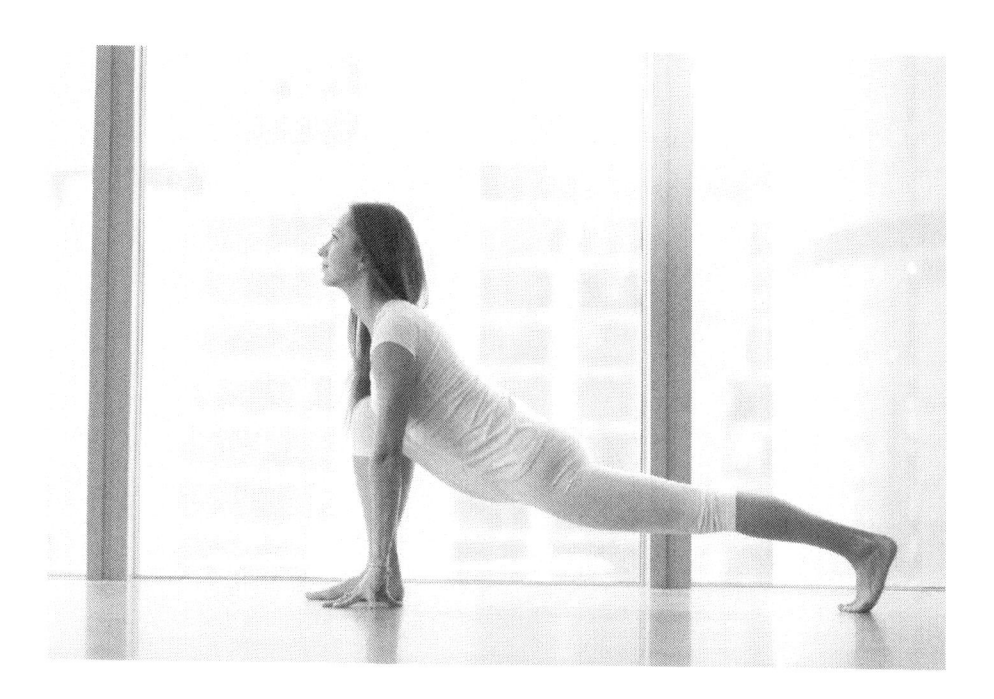

Instructions

1. Go into downward facing dog pose, in which your palms and feet are on the floor with your legs and hands completely stretched, making you resemble an inverted 'V'.
2. Bring your right foot forward and place it on the outside of the right hand.
3. Lengthen your spine and stretch your chest forward. Raise the left heel off the floor so the toes are tucked in, pointing forward.
4. Look straight ahead.
5. Remain in the pose for 30 seconds.
6. Bring the right leg back, and straighten your arms and legs so you are now in downward dog pose again.
7. Repeat the same steps with the other leg.
8. You may rest in child's pose if necessary.

Benefits
- Opens the hips
- Stretches the spine
- Tones and strengthens the back
- Opens the chest
- Stimulates the abdominal organs, improves digestion, and relieves gas
- Strengthens the shoulders, arms, and legs
- Calms the mind

Caution
Those with a lower back injury or sciatica should refrain from practicing this pose.

Yoga for Meditation

Here is the perfect way to complete your yoga session for the day. While meditation can also be done as an individual practice without combining it with yoga, performing yoga prepares your body, mind, and soul for your meditation practice. Yoga strengthens your body, stimulates your chakras (or energy centers) and calms your mind. There cannot be a better preparation for meditation.

Below, we show you some of the best ways to perform meditation. Lotus pose is considered the best pose for meditation. Instructions for this pose are given under the 'Headache' chapter.

The Accomplished Pose

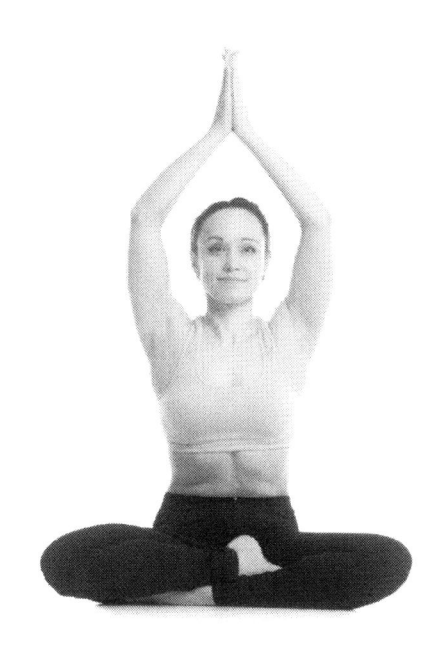

Instructions
1. Sit on the mat with your legs outstretched.
2. Draw your left foot in, and place the heel near the perineum.
3. Bend your right leg, and place your right foot over the left foot, sliding the toes between the thigh and calf muscles of the left leg. The ankles should be in contact.
4. Place your palms on your knees in chin mudra. You can also stretch your arms over your head and hold the palms together.
5. Remain in the pose as long as you feel the need.

Benefits
- Easy, important pose for meditation
- Keeps the spine straight
- Strengthens the nervous system

Caution
Avoid practicing this pose if you have sciatica.

Auspicious Pose

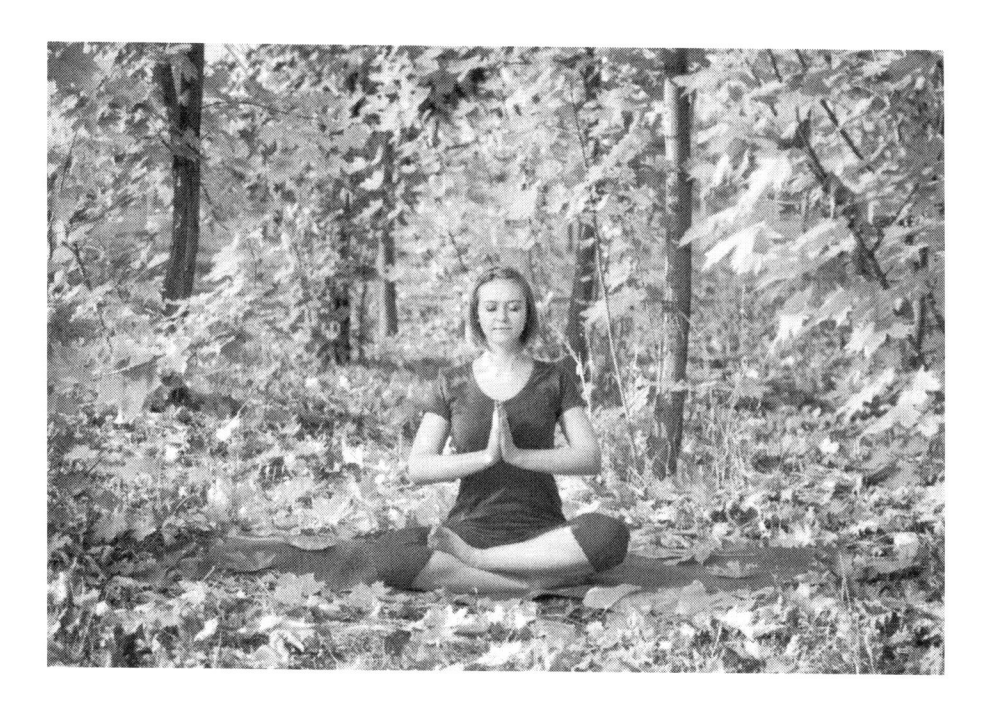

Instructions
1. Sit on the yoga mat. Keep your legs outstretched.
2. Bend your left leg. Place the left foot against the inner thigh of your right leg.
3. Draw your right leg in and slide the right foot between the thigh and calf muscles of the left leg.
4. Hold the toes of the left foot and draw the foot up to position it between the calf muscles and thigh of the right leg.
5. Keep the knees firmly on the ground.
6. Lengthen your spine.
7. Place your hands on your knees in chin mudra.
8. Focus on your breath.

Benefits
- Stretches and tones the spine
- Rejuvenates the nervous system
- Relieves leg pain
- Promotes focus
- Calms the mind

Caution
Those with sciatica or a knee injury should avoid practicing this pose.

Anal Lock

Mula Bandha is one of the three main Bandhas, meaning 'locks'.

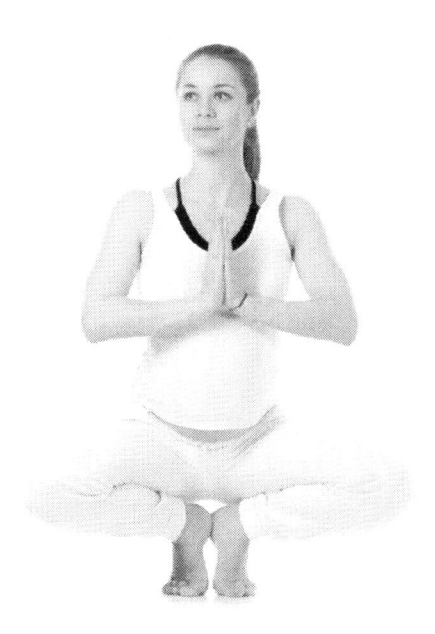

Instructions
1. Sit in accomplished pose. You can also sit on your heels, keeping the knees apart.
2. Keep the spine erect.
3. Contract your pelvic floor muscles and engage the lower abdominal muscles. In the initial stages of the practice you will have to contract your anus and genitals. With practice, you will relax these muscles and engage the perineum, the space between the anus and genitals.
4. Inhale. Hold the breath while contracting the muscles.
5. Remain in the lock as long as you are comfortable.
6. Release the lock and breathe normally.

Benefits
- Strengthens the core
- Energizes the body
- Builds stamina
- Relieves constipation
- Improves digestion
- Calms the autonomic nervous system
- Postpones symptoms of aging
- Helps regulate menstrual cycles
- Relieves depression
- Spiritually, it awakens the inner consciousness and elevates your state of mind to a higher level.

Caution
Pregnant women should avoid practicing this pose, as should those with hernia.

Yogic Sleep

Yoga Nidra is one of the ideal practices to perform towards the end of your yogic session.

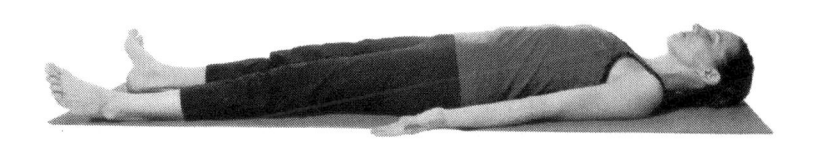

Instructions

1. Lie down in corpse pose, in which you keep your legs stretched, hands by your sides, and the entire body relaxed.
2. Close your eyes.
3. Take a few slow, deep breaths.
4. Think about your intention for the meditation. Feel the intention embrace your body, mind, and soul. After being conscious of your intention for some time, relax your mind and shift your focus to your body.
5. Start with focusing on your right foot. Mentally observe and relax the foot.
6. Move your attention to your right knee and thigh. Observe the parts of the leg as a whole. Repeat the same for the left leg.

7. Now, take your attention from the legs and move it to every part of the body, until you reach the crown of your head.
8. Mentally observe the sensations your body is experiencing.
9. Relax deeply in stillness. Meditate in the relaxed state as long as you need.
10. When you are completely relaxed and ready to come out of meditation, focus on how calm your body is. Mentally observe your surroundings.
11. After a couple of minutes or more, roll over to your right and remain in that position for few minutes. The concept behind remaining on the right side is to make your breath flow through your left nostril, thereby cooling the body.
12. Place your left palm on the floor in front of your body, and pressing the palm to the ground, get up and sit.
13. Open your eyes slowly.

Benefits

- Sends you into a state of deep relaxation
- Rejuvenates the body and mind
- Calms the nervous system
- Improves the quality of your thoughts and actions
- Relieves stress
- Cures insomnia
- Supports your health
- Improves focus
- Promotes awareness
- Connects you with your inner self
- Promotes a sense of calm

Yoga Sequences for Beginners

Incorporating yoga sequences in your yoga session optimizes the benefits of yoga. Performing yoga poses in a flowing style keeps your focus on your practice, and helps keep you interested. Because of the various poses in a sequence, you get a better workout. Hold each pose briefly, and find your breath before moving on to the next one.

You can get creative and come up with your own yoga sequence. Here is some simple sequences to get you going.

Sun Salutation

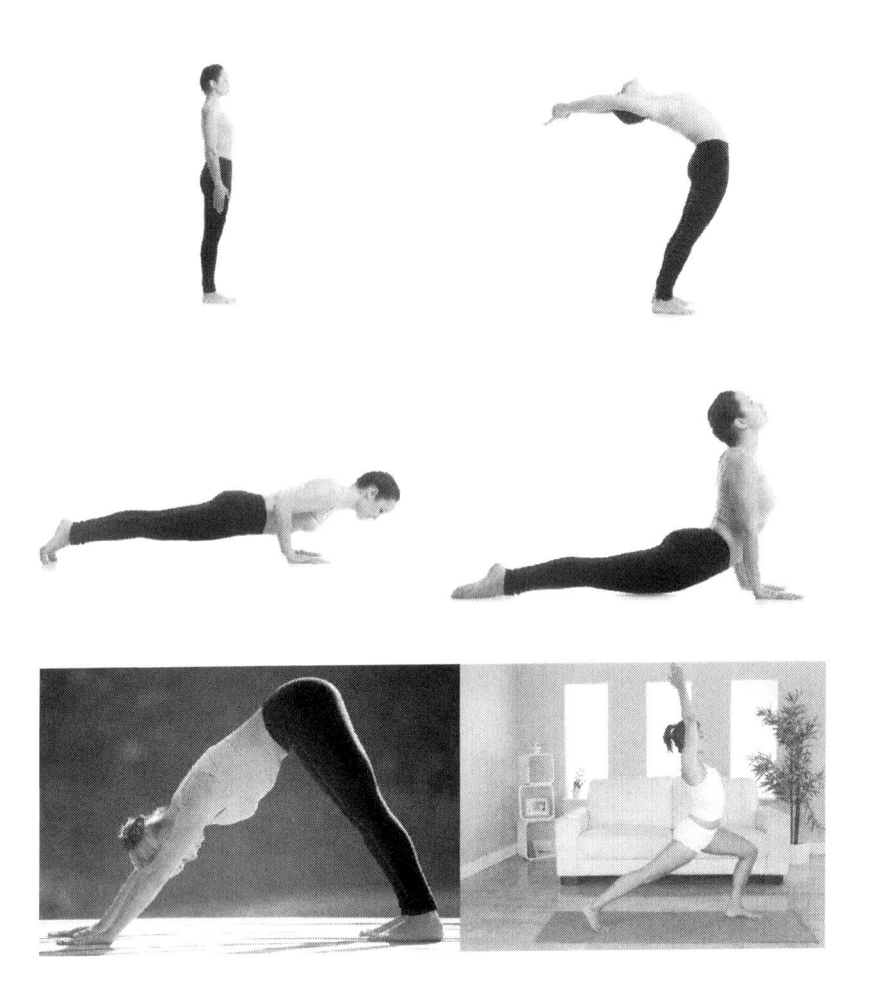

1. Start in mountain pose, keeping your palms together as in prayer.
2. Inhale, stretch your arms over your head, and arch your back, assuming half wheel pose.
3. Exhale as you bend forward, with your hands reaching for the floor on the outer side of the feet, as in standing forward bend. You may also bend your knees.

4. Inhale as you stretch your right leg backwards. Tuck in your toes so your foot is straight. Exhale.
5. Inhale as you bring the left leg back to place it closer to the right foot. Now your legs will be straight and your body will be in one straight line from back to heels.
6. Exhale and bend your elbows to bring your torso closer to the ground. Your body will be parallel to the floor in four-limbed staff pose.
7. Place your chin, chest, knees, and toes on the floor, keeping your hips lifted.
8. Inhale, lift your torso up, and arch your back, straightening your hands. Lift your knees. Now you will be on your palms and the front sides of your feet in upward facing dog pose.
9. Exhale. Raise your hips high and place your feet on the ground, stretching your arms and legs in downward dog pose.
10. Inhale as you bring your right leg forward to place it on the inner side of your right palm, as in high lunge pose.
11. Exhale, bring your left leg forward, and place the left foot close to the right foot. Stretch your knees and assume standing forward bend.
12. Inhale, lift your torso and your arms over your head and draw the palms down in front of your chest as in prayer.

Standing Yoga Sequence

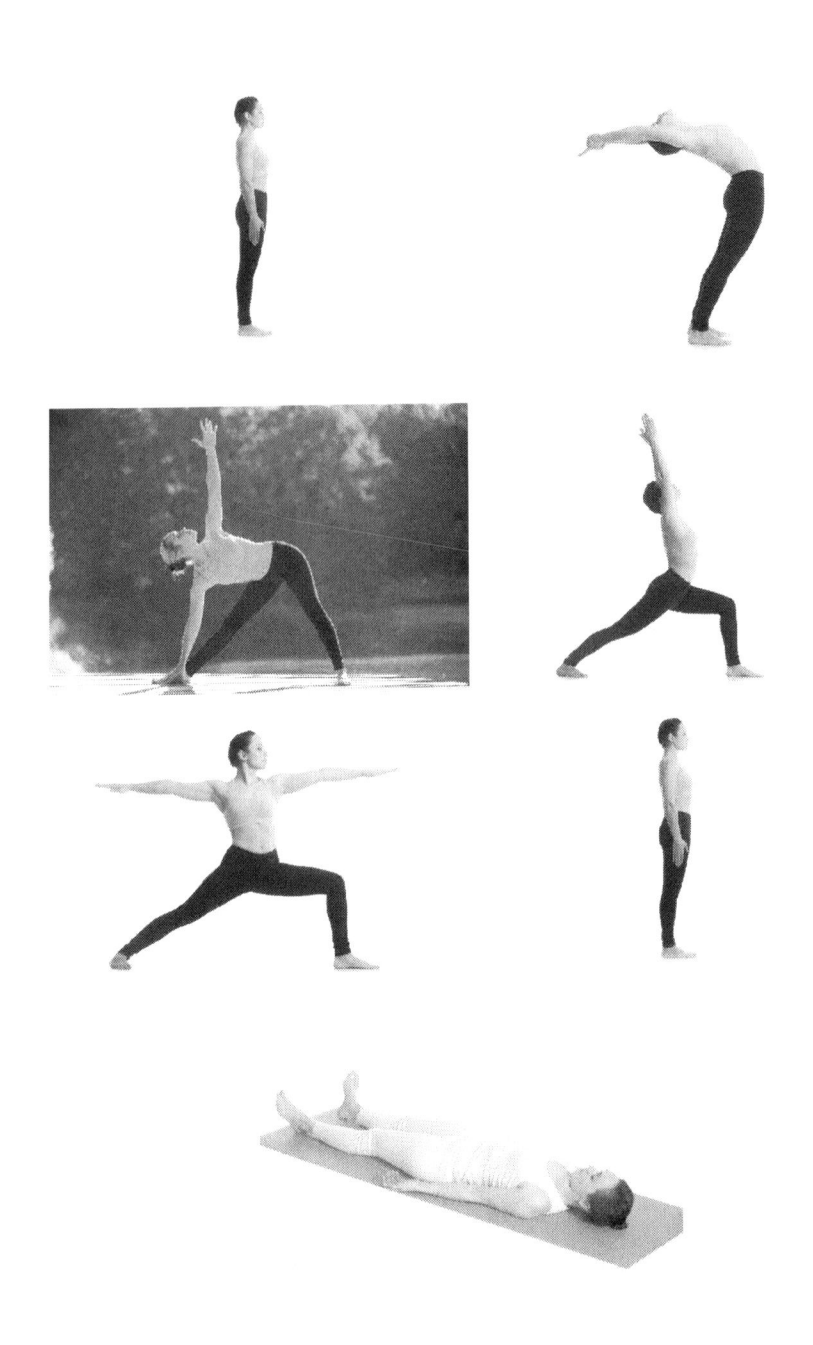

1. Start in mountain pose.
2. Inhale and bend backwards, to go into half wheel pose.
3. Exhale as you come forward, and bend to perform standing forward bend.
4. Place your legs few feet apart, and stretch your hands sideways. Bend towards your right and place your right palm on the floor, close to your right foot, in extended triangle pose. Repeat the same thing on the other side.
5. From triangle pose, rise and stand straight. Twist your torso to your right and place your right hand on the outer side of the left foot.
6. Turn your right foot towards your right at a 90 degree angle, and your left foot slightly towards your right. Turn your torso to your right, stretch your hands sideways at shoulder-height and over your head. Bend your right knee until the knee is in line with your right ankle. Bring the palms together over your head in warrior I pose.
7. From warrior I pose, bring the palms sideways and stretch the arms over the legs. Turn your head forwards, in warrior II pose.
8. Release warrior II pose, and bring your feet together and your hands to your sides in mountain pose.
9. Relax in corpse pose.

Seated Yoga Sequence

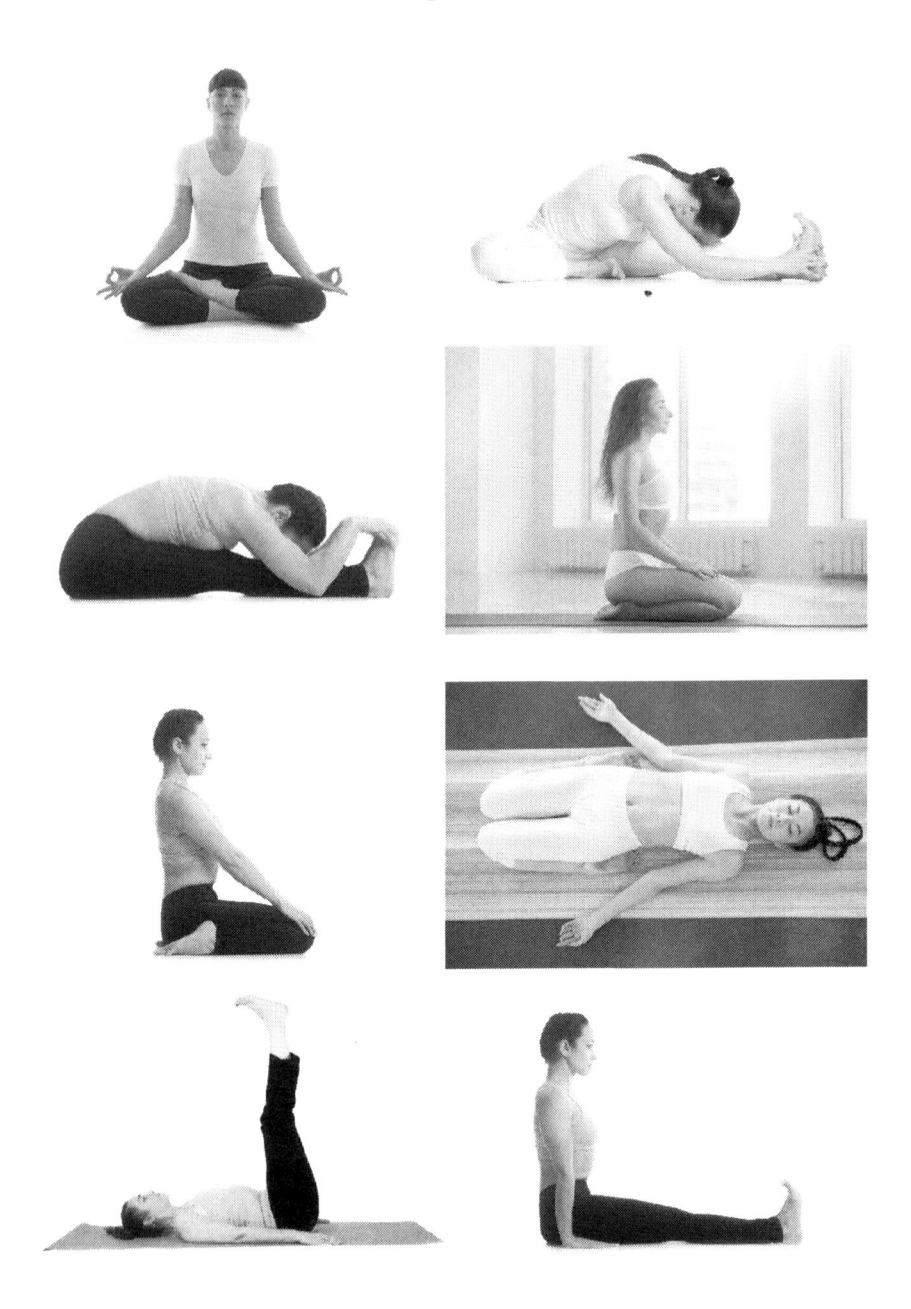

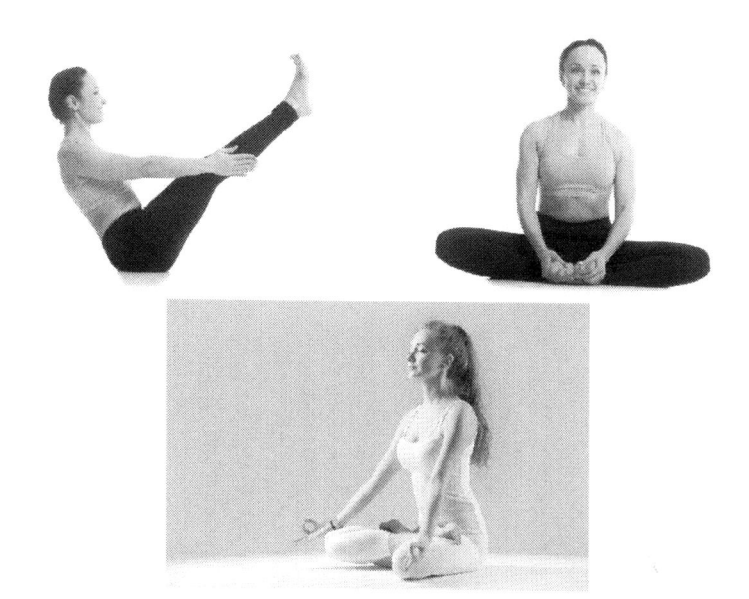

1. Start in easy pose, in which you sit on the floor, crossing your legs with your palms on your knees.
2. Stretch your right leg forward, and do head to knee pose.
3. Repeat head to knee pose, extending the left leg.
4. Now, stretch both the legs and perform seated forward bend.
5. Bend your legs to take a kneeling position. Lift your buttocks, bring your big toes together, and sit in the space between the heels, in thunderbolt pose.
6. Lift your buttocks, place your legs hip-width apart and sit down in the space, keeping your lower legs close to the outer side of your thighs, in hero pose.
7. From hero pose, lean back to perform reclining hero pose.
8. Release your legs and stretch them forward. Place your hands by your sides and perform half plough pose, keeping your legs at 45 degrees.
9. Lift your legs straight so they are perpendicular to the floor.
10. Place your legs back, get up, and sit in staff pose (p19).

11. From staff pose, lift your legs up and balance on the sit bones to perform boat pose.
12. Place your legs on the floor, bring the feet together, and perform bound angle pose.
13. Stretch your legs, and place the feet on the opposite thighs. Sit straight, and keep your palms on the knees in chin mudra, for lotus pose.

Supine Sequence

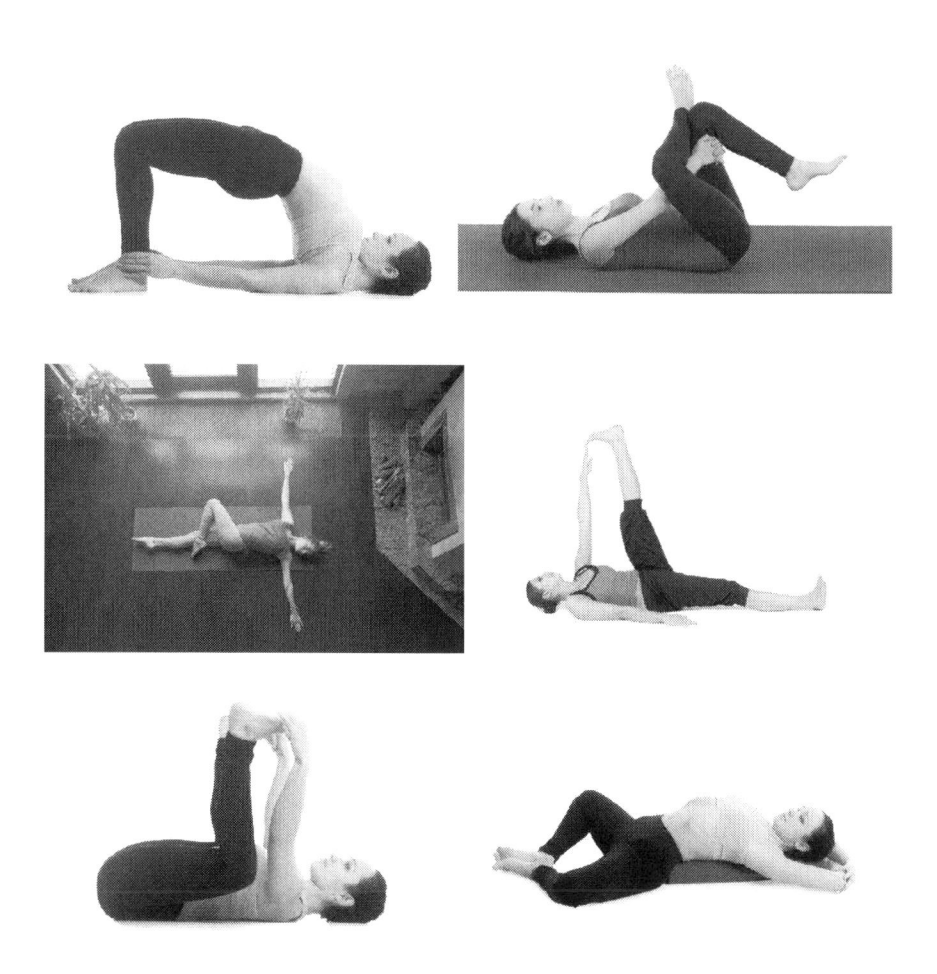

1. Lie down on the floor, stretch your legs out, and place your hands by your sides.
2. Bend your legs and place your feet on the floor, keeping the ankles aligned with your knees vertically. Lift your hips off the floor, and perform bridge pose.
3. From bridge pose, perform eye of the needle pose.
4. Release the pose, and stretch your legs forward. Relax and twist your torso to your left, placing your right foot outside the left thigh to perform supine spinal twist.

5. After performing supine spinal twist, stretch your legs and keep your hands by your sides. Bend your right leg and draw the right foot towards your chest. Hold the big toe of the right foot with your right hand, and stretch the leg straight in reclining hand-to-big-toe pose. Repeat the same with the other leg. Stretch your legs.
6. Bend your legs and bring your knees forward. Hold your feet to go into happy baby pose.
7. Place your legs back on the floor, bring the soles of the feet together, and perform reclining bound angle pose.

Breathing and Meditation

Breathing practice is an integral part of yoga. The breathing techniques of yoga promote physical and psychological health. Pranayama, meaning breathing techniques, are performed after performing asanas. Pranayama prepares you for meditation, a practice that involves attaining inner peace.

Benefits of Pranayama

Benefits of pranayama include:

- Improves respiratory function
- Improves blood circulation
- Lowers high blood pressure
- Supports heart health
- Improves digestion
- Promotes longevity
- Calms the nerves
- Relieves muscular tension
- Relieves stress and depression
- Sets the stage for meditation

Types of Pranayama for Beginners

Out of the various pranayama types, here are the best for beginners.

1) Skull Shining Breath Technique / Kapalabhati Pranayama

Instructions
1. Sit in easy pose or thunderbolt pose (or any other pose that is comfortable to you). Your spine should be straight. Place your hands on your knees.
2. Focus on your lower belly. You can also place your hands on your lower belly so you stay focused.
3. Inhale deeply through your nostrils.
4. Pressing the lower belly with your hands, exhale quickly.
5. Your quick exhalation should be followed by passive inhalation.
6. Repeat for one minute.

Benefits
- Energizes the body
- Improves brain function
- Cleanses the lungs and improves respiratory function
- Strengthens the abdominal muscles

Note
Beginners can start with a few rounds per day. The contractions can be gradually increased to doing up to 100 inhalations and exhalations per minute.

Caution

Do not force yourself to perform beyond your limits. It is absolutely essential that you increase the number of contractions gradually.

Those with high blood pressure, hernia, or heart conditions should not practice this pranayama. Pregnant women should also refrain from practicing this pranayama.

2) Alternate Nostril Breathing / Nadi Shodhana

Instructions
1. Sit in a comfortable pose.
2. Perform mrigi mudra with your right hand, in which you stretch the thumb, ring, and little fingers of your right hand, folding the index and middle fingers.
3. Place your right thumb on the right nostril.
4. Inhale deeply through your left nostril, and then close the left nostril with your ring finger and little finger.
5. Exhale through the right nostril. Keep the right nostril open after the exhalation, to inhale.
6. Close the right nostril now, and exhale through the left. This is one cycle.
7. Do five cycles to start. As you advance in practice you can increase the number of repetitions.

Benefits
- Balances the right and left hemispheres of the brain
- Lowers the heart rate
- Improves focus
- Relieves stress
- Supports deep meditation

Note
Those with injury to the neck or shoulders can use a prop to support the right arm.

Caution
Those with high blood pressure should perform the pranayama under expert guidance.

Practicing Pranayama and Meditation

The ideal time to practice pranayama and meditation is in the early hours of the day. While meditation can also be performed in the night, performing in the quiet of the morning when the mind is fresh from a good sleep works best.

Both pranayama and meditation should be performed only on an empty stomach. Meditation can be performed in any of the meditation poses given in the earlier chapter.

Choose a quiet place for your practice. Keep the room well ventilated.

Set a particular time of the day for your practice. It helps you to be regular and consistent.

Parting Words

While the poses are beginners' poses, they may not all be easy for those with lower flexibility levels. As you well know, practice makes perfect. All you need to do is keep working at improving the postures by practicing regularly. Never push beyond your limits, as such attempts may result in injury.

We recommend you practice yoga for at least three months consistently before you evaluate the results of yoga practice.

We wish you the best in your efforts on the yoga mat.

Namasté